Notes on Minor Surgery

By

Dr. Debasish Kundu Ph.D.

Guided & Edited by

Dr. A.K. Banerjee

M.B.B.S., M.D. (U.S.A.)

Originals

Delhi

First Published 2017

Illustrations: Author/Editor/other open sources

ISBN 13: 978-81-8454-191-5

ISBN 10: 81-8454-191-0

Published By

Originals

A-6, Second Floor, Nimri Commercial Centre,

Ashok Vihar Phase-4, Delhi - 110 052 (India)

Tel.: +91 11 2730 2453 Fax: 011 4706 1936

Website: www.Lppindia.com, e-mail: info@Lppindia.com

Printed At

D K Fine Art Press P Ltd.

Delhi-110052

PRINTED IN INDIA

Contents

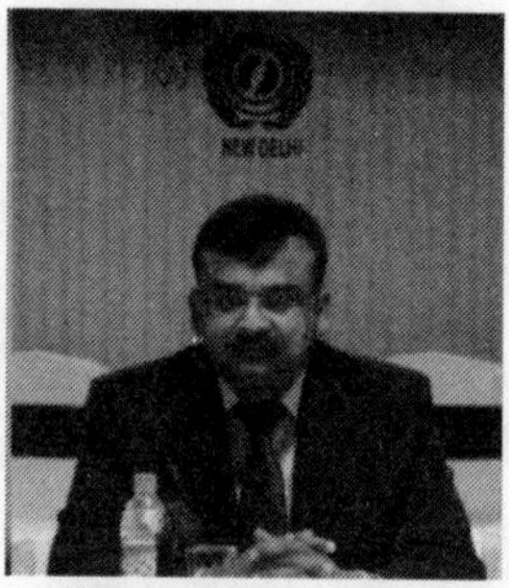

Foreword

I am pleased to have the opportunity to write foreword for the book of Notes on Minor Surgery which is written by Dr. Debasish Kundu for ADEH students. Because I have a dream for all my Electro Homoeopathic practitioners that one day they must get an official Certificate from any Government Agency and I am happy to say that Maharashtra is the First State in India to offer an Official Electro Homoeopathy Certificate which is being awarded by the Government Agency. Also I have some friends who helped me to fulfill my dream to introduce a Government recognised ADVANCE DIPLOMA IN ELECTRO HOMOEOPATHY (ADEH) course in Maharashtra.

When word comes "ADVANCED" means something new and scientific, so while reading the contents of the book, I found something new and advanced. Since long time Dr. Kundu is writing books on different subjects which are very easy to understand and rich in contents, so I believe this book will help all the Students, Practitioners & Lovers of Electro-Homoeopathy besides students in perusing ADEH examination which contains the study material mentioned in Syllabus by MSBVE, Mumbai. This entire course material will help to improve the knowledge in Electro Homoeopathy subject.

Dr. Trideep Guha
BPTH, MD (ECH) MBA, Ph.D., MRCE (USA)
Chairman
Educational & Medical/Paramedical Council of India
Executive Member:
Paramedical Syllabus Committee,
MSBVEE, Mumbai (Govt. of Maharashtra)

Email id
drtrideep.g@gmail.com, empci@hotmail.com
Visit us at :
www.empci.com

Published By

Originals

A-6, Second Floor, Nimri Commercial Centre,
Ashok Vihar Phase-4, Delhi - 110 052 (India)
Tel.: +91 11 2730 2453 Fax: 011 4706 1936
Website: www.Lppindia.com
e-mail: info@Lppindia.com

In Association with

ADEH PRACTISIONERS ASSOCIATION MAHARASHTRA

N-123, Second floor, Infront of Devanjali flats,
Reshimbag, City & District : Nagpur
State : Maharashtra Country : INDIA
Phone : +91-712-2700606, +91-712-2700651, +91-712-2700777

Preface

This notebook describes a limited number of surgical procedures. They have been chosen as appropriate for the doctors who does not have a full-fledged surgical training alike the MBBS students, hence all the procedures included in this small notebook are considered essential for saving life, alleviating pain, preventing the development of serious complications, or stabilizing a patient's condition pending referral. Operations that require specialist skills have been avoided, and simple but standard surgical techniques have been included. However, certain procedures that may appear technically difficult but may offer the best chance of saving a patient's life are carefully chosen and included. Clinical examination forms an important part in surgery, hence, an outline of discussion of various cases are covered which are commonly encountered in clinical practice.

The aim of this book is to assist the doctors who might undertake minor surgery in their practices. It is intended to present a comprehensive, clear and concise text with easy to follow illustrations. No surgery can be considered "minor", it requires a thorough knowledge of anatomy and basic surgical procedures besides technical skills. Careful observation and planning is needed at all stages. The Practitioner should bear the attitude of Arjuna and not Abhimanyu. Every effort should be made to keep the tissue structure intact so far as possible to help early recovery and healing. Importance should always be given to sterility of instruments and general health condition of the patients besides anaesthesia(if the blood which oozes is bright red while making an incision, then the anaesthesia has been done satisfactorily and if the blood is dark red then there's something not correct). Facilities should also be available to deal with any complications and emergencies which may occur.

We are thankful to Ms. Rashleen Kaur MBBS student who assisted us in preparing the manuscript.

Dr. Debasish Kundu
Dr. A.K. Banerjee

Part I

1

Acharya Sushruta

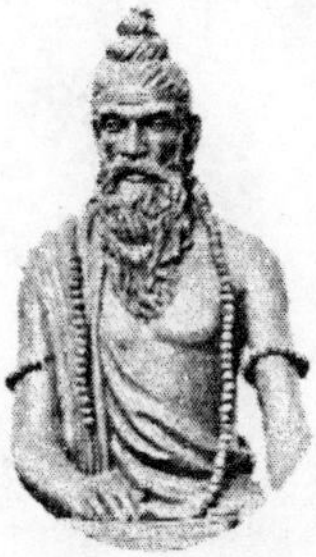

Acharya Sushruta born to sage Vishwamitra, Sushruta is the father of surgery.

During 1500 BC, he and health scientists of his time conducted complicated surgeries like cesareans, cataract, artificial limbs, Rhinoplasty (restoration of a damaged nose), 12 types of fractures, 6 types of dislocations, urinary stones and even plastic surgery and brain surgery.

Usage of anesthesia was well known in ancient India.

He is the author of the book "*Sushruta Samhita*", in which he describes over 300 surgical procedures and 125 surgical Instruments to drain fluids, to remove kidney stones, to sew: up wounds and to perform plastic surgery, including scalpels, lancets, needles, Cathers and rectal speculums; mostly designed from the jaws of animals and birds.

Acharya Sudhruta details the first ever surgery procedures in "*Sushruta Samhita*," a unique encyclopedia of surgery. He is venerated as the father of plastic surgery and the science of anesthesia.

When surgery was in its infancy in Europe, Sushruta was performing Rhinoplasty (restoration of a damaged nose) and other critical operations.

In the "*Sushruta Samhita*," he describes treatment for twelve types of fractures and six types of dislocations. His details on human embryology are simply amazing.

He has also described a number of stitching methods: the use of horse's hair as thread and fibers of bark in the "*Sushruta Samhita*,".

2

Basic Surgical Procedures

Surgical operations must satisfy three basic conditions: the wound must be inflicted without pain; haemorrhage must be arrested; and the wound must heal. It is especially the ability to ensure wound healing, by means of aseptic treatment, that has given impetus to modern surgery. Indeed, the necessity for asepsis regulates the conduct of surgeons, the "ritual" of operation, the form of instruments, and even hospital design and construction to such an extent that it is often taken for granted. Yet an understanding of the practical details of this system is imperative for any surgeon.

The patient's stay in hospital before an operation should be as short as possible.

Therefore, any tests and treatment that could prolong the preoperative stay beyond 24 hours should be carried out as outpatient services, if possible. Before the operation, correct gross malnutrition, treat serious bacterial infection, investigate and correct gross anaemia, and control diabetes. As a routine, measure the patient's haemoglobin level and test the urine for sugar and protein.

The patient should bathe the night before an elective operation. Hair in the operative site should not be removed unless it will interfere with the surgical procedure. If it must be removed, clipping is preferable to shaving (which can damage the skin) and should be done as close as possible to the time of operation.

Just before the operation, wash the area around and including the operative site, and prepare the skin with antiseptic solution, starting in the centre and moving out to the periphery (Fig. 1.1). This area should be large enough to include the entire incision and an adjacent working area, so that you can manoeuvre during the operation without touching unprepared skin. Ethanol 70% (by volume) is recommended as an antiseptic, except for delicate skin, such as that of the genitalia and near the eye, and for children; 1% cetrimide (10 g/litre) is an alternative, as is 2.5% iodine in ethanol (25 gllitre).

For surgeries involving an incision and requiring the use of the operating room, cover the patient with sterile drapes, leaving no part uncovered except the. operative field and those areas necessary for the maintenance of anaesthesia.

Many important procedures can be performed under local anaesthesia.

In most outpatient procedures, local or field block anaesthesia will be sufficient but general anaesthesia, including ketamine, may be necessary in children and should be available.

Irrespective of the seriousness of a wound, give initial management priority to the airway, breathing and circulation.

Good lighting and basic instruments are important for adequate wound examination and management.

Work efficiently to avoid prolonging the operation unnecessarily; the risk of infection increases with time.

Universal precautions are necessary to avoid the transmission of the HIV, hepatitis, Ebola and other viruses.

Clear the operative field of devitalized tissue and foreign material.

While not a substitute for appropriate haemostasis, placement of a drain is an option if a wound is oozing; the collection of fluid and blood leads to increased risk of infection and delayed healing.

Minimize dead space when closing a wound.

Lacerations may be associated with neurovascular or other serious injury; a complete examination is required to identify the injuries that are not immediately obvious.

Minor problems are important because mismanagement can lead to major detrimental consequences.

The removal of a foreign body may be urgent, as in the case of airway compromise or unnecessary, as in the case of some deep metal fragments.

Foreign body removal may be difficult or time- consuming; the patient should therefore be anaesthetized.

X-ray or fluoroscopy is recommended for the removal of radiopaque objects.

Foreign bodies in the cranium, chest or abdomen or in close proximity to vital structures must be removed in an operating room with a team prepared to manage possible complications.

Failure of a superficial infection to respond to medical management may be due to resistance to the antibiotic or to the presence of an abscess cavity.

If an abscess cavity is identified, drain it with a surgical incision.

Adequate surgical drainage requires anaesthesia to ensure that all parts of the abscess cavity are exposed.

If there is doubt about the diagnosis of abscess, confirm the presence of pus with needle aspiration.

Prepare the skin and give adequate anaesthesia.

Perform the preliminary aspiration using an 18 gauge or larger needle to confirm the presence of pus.

Introduce the tip of a pair of artery forceps into the abscess cavity and open the jaws.

Explore the cavity with a finger to break down all the septa.

Extend the incision if necessary for complete drainage.

Excise benign lesions for treatment and confirmation of the diagnosis.

Establish the diagnosis of malignant disease by biopsy before beginning definitive treatment.

Obtain material for histological examination with:

- Incision biopsies when part of the tumour is removed.
- Excision biopsies when the whole tumour is removed with a margin of surrounding normal tissues.
- Needle biopsies when a core of tissue is removed.

Obtain material for cytolological examination with a fine needle aspiration; false negative results occur if the biopsy does not include the lesion or if the lesion is necrotic.

Necrosis occurs with the use of electro-cautery, therefore excise the tumour with a scalpel.

Sterilization

The methods of sterilization in wide use are autoclaving, exposure to dry heat, and treatment with chemical antiseptics.

Sterilization should be largely based on autoclaving. For efficient use, an autoclave demands a trained operator in regular practice and depends heavily on good maintenance. Most autoclaves in current use are too large and too complicated, and carry high maintenance costs. It is therefore hoped that more effort will be put into developing smaller and simpler autoclaves that require little maintenance and are possibly solar-powered, especially for use in isolated rural hospitals in developing countries.

The basic operational criteria for an autoclave are steam at 100.0 kPa (750 mmHg) above atmospheric pressure and a temperature of 120°C maintained for 15 min (or for 30 min for packs). Appropriate indicators must be used each time to show that sterilization has been accomplished. At the end of the procedure, the outsides of the packs of instruments should have no wet spots, and the moisture retained by each pack should not cause more than a 3% increase in its weight.

Anaesthesia

It is the anaesthetist's responsibility to provide safe and effective anaesthesia for the patient. The anaesthetic of choice for any given procedure will depend on the anaesthetist's training and experience, the range of equipment and drugs available, and the clinical situation.

Respecting Tissue Integrity

The surgical team should strive to handle tissues gently, to prevent bleeding, to minimize dead space and the amount of devitalized tissue and foreign material in the wound, and to work efficiently to avoid prolonging the operation unnecesarily. Plan the incision to give adequate exposure. Incise the skin with bold sweeps of the belly of the knife, while stretching the skin between the thumb and fingers of the other hand (Fig. 1.1). Control initial oozing of blood from the cut surfaces by pressure over gauze. Individual bleeding vessels may be caught in fine forceps and twisted off or ligated with fine catgut or fine thread (Fig. 1.2). Cut the ligature short. As a routine, use a reef knot, but make a triple knot or a surgeon's knot if additional security is required. Avoid diathermy near the skin. Similarly deepen the wound to reach the target organ, making sure that the wound is laid open along its whole length. A clean knife is commonly used to gain access to a body cavity, for example for incising the peritoneum.

Close the operation wound in layers with catgut, thread, or nylon (but avoid thread in potentially contaminated wounds because it can form a focus for infection). Use

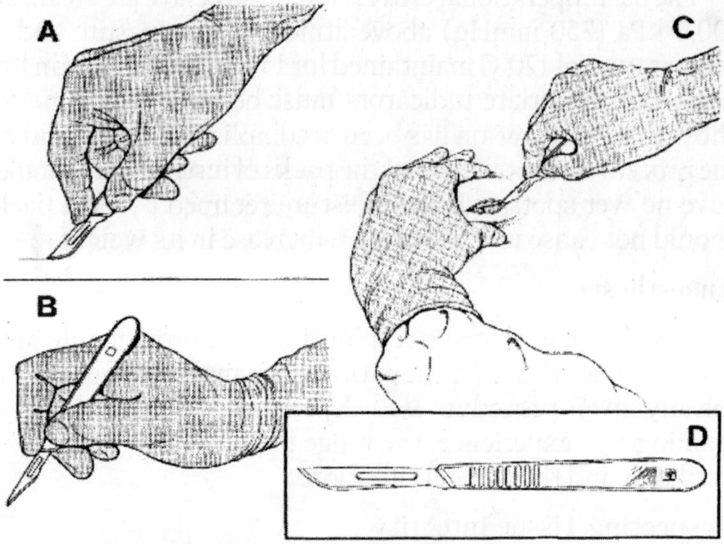

Fig. 1.1

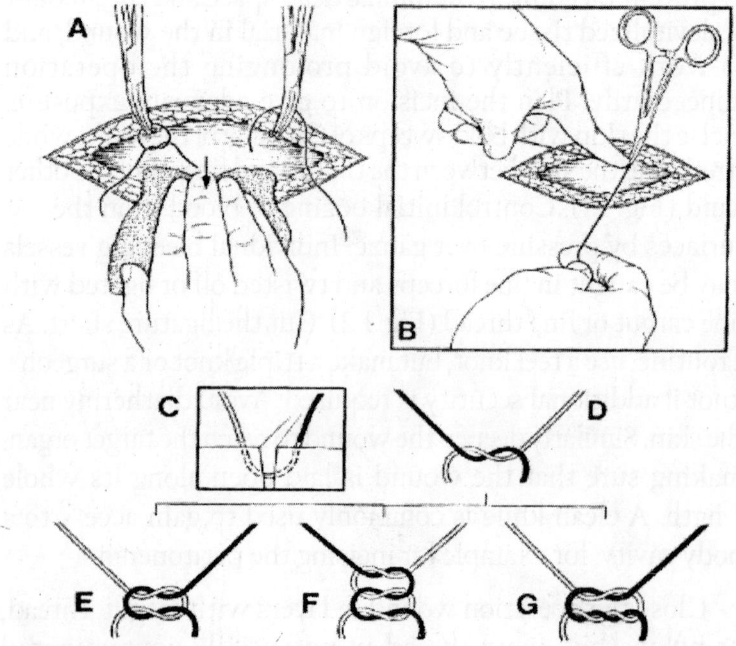

Fig. 1.2

different types of sutures as appropriate, for example simple, interrupted, continuous, mattress, or purse-string. Aim to bring the wound edges together loosely, but without gaps, taking a "bite" of about 1 cm of tissue on either side and leaving an interval of 1 cm between each stitch (Fig. 1.3 A-D). Remember that a "suspect" (possibly contaminated) or grossly contaminated wound is best left open and lightly packed with plenty of dry gauze, with sutures inserted for delayed primary closure after 2-5 days (Fig. 1.3 E, F).

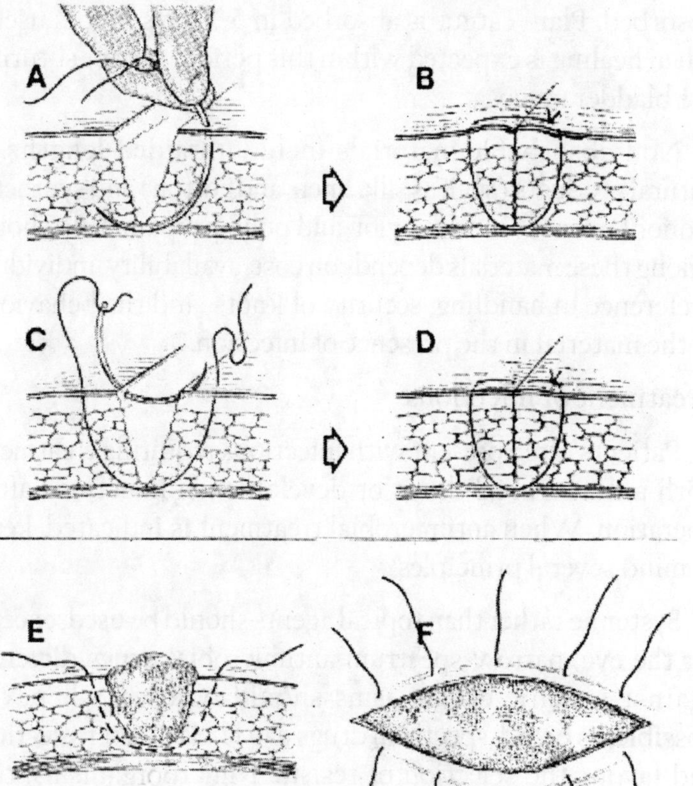

Fig. 1.3 A-F

Suture Materials

Sutures and ligatures consist of absorbable or non-absorbable materials. Catgut remains the most popular absorbable material because of its pliability and superior handling qualities. Chromic catgut lasts for 2 or 3 weeks in the tissues and is excellent for ligatures and for approximating tissues, though it is no longer used for closing abdominal wounds and in other situations where prolonged support is needed, because of the rapid loss of tensile strength as it is absorbed. Plain catgut is absorbed in 5-7 days, but is useful when healing is expected within this period, and for suturing the bladder mucosa.

Non-absorbable materials include braided lengths of natural products (such as silk, linen, and cotton) and synthetic monofilaments (such as nylon and poly- propamide). Choice among these materials depends on cost, availability, individual preference in handling, security of knots, and the behaviour of the material in the presence of infection.

Treatment of infections

Patients often present with infections requiring treatment with antimicrobial drugs or develop such infections after operation. When antimicrobial treatment is indicated, keep in mind several principles:

Systemic rather than topical agents should be used, except for the eye; narrow-spectrum antimicrobial drugs directed against specific organ- isms should be used whenever possible, as broad-spectrum drugs can lead to superinfection and favour the selection of resistant microorganisms; the choice of a particular agent from a broad group of antimicrobial drugs should depend on the target microorganism, if known, and its drug sensitivity, and on factors such as the drug's antimicrobial spectrum, record of use in the clinic, safety, efficacy, and potential to favour the selection of resistant organisms; cost should determine the choice of drug when microbiological, pharmacological, and other relevant properties are similar for several agents; antimicrobial treatment should be discontinued as soon as the patient's clinical condition permits.

Parenteral antimicrobial prophylaxis should not be routine, but is recommended for operations associated with a high risk of infection, for example bowel resection. It is also recommended for operations after which infection, although not a frequent problem, can have severe or life-threatening consequences (for example, craniotomy). In addition, antimicrobial prophylaxis is essential for patients with valvular heart disease, who are at risk of developing bacterial endocarditis as a result of transient bacteraemia from instrumentation in the mouth or other parts of the body.

Wound Care

Generally, do not close wounds by primary suture if they are or may be contaminated, and do not touch an open wound directly with bare, unsterilized hands. A repaired wound can be regarded as sealed after 24 hours, and dressings may then be changed without sterile gloves but should not be touched directly.

Remove dressings over closed wounds if they become wet or if the patient shows signs or symptoms suggestive of infection, for example fever or unusual wound pain. After removing the dressing, inspect the wound for signs of infection and sample any discharge for bacteriological examination.

Primary Care of Wounds of the Face

Although the doctors at the private clinics are usually expected to treat patients with small facial wounds, patients with large wounds or wounds associated with tissue loss should normally be referred for specialized care.

If referral is necessary, first ensure that it is safe to transport the patient. Maintain a clear airway, if necessary by tracheal intubation or tracheostomy. Arrest any obvious bleeding. If immediate referral is impossible, confine treatment of extensive wounds to thorough cleaning of the wound area and tethering of the wound edges using local skin landmarks as a guide for alignment.

General Principles

When you are treating facial wounds, whether minor or serious, your priority is to keep the patient's airway clear at all times. Remember too that a severe facial injury may be associated with other injuries, which may also require your attention.

The choice of anaesthetic for the patient will normally depend on the nature of the injuries, but general anaesthesia is preferable in children. Use good lighting and fine instruments when examining and treating wounds of the face; ophthalmic instruments are ideal for this. Unless the wound is near the eyes, clean it with soap and water, while protecting the patient's eyes, and then irrigate it with saline. Make every attempt to preserve tissue, especially skin, but remove all foreign material and all obviously devitalized tissue. A small, soft brush will facilitate this process.

Always administer tetanus toxoid. Cellulitis, a potentially serious complication, can be prevented by meticulous surgery and by prophylactic benzylpenicillin 600 mg (106 units) given twice a day intramuscularly.

Equipments for Minor Surgery (Fig.0.1-0.5):

Olsen Hager Needle Holder 14cm

Mayo Scissors 15cm TC

Kelly Forceps 14cm Straight

Kelly Forceps 14cm Curved

Adson Forceps 12cm

Adson Forceps 1:2 12cm

Mosquito Forceps 12.5cm Straight

Mosquito Forceps 12.5cm Curved

Iris Scissors 11.5cm

Spencer Scissors 11cm

Scalpel Handle # 3

05 Blades for Scalpel Handle # 3

Scalpel Handle # 4

05 Blades for Scalpel Handle # 4

Dressing Forceps 16cm

Ophthalmic Instruments:

Eyelid speculum, 1

Eyelid retractors, 2

Forceps, 0.5 mm or 0.9 mm, toothed, 1

Forceps, 0.5 mm or 0.9 mm, non-toothed, 1

Straight ring scissors, 1 pair

Small needle holder, 1

Scalpel handle with No. 11 blade, 1

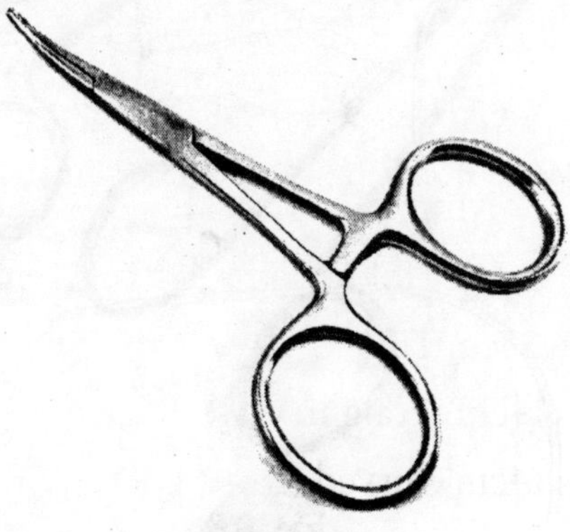

Fig. 0.1

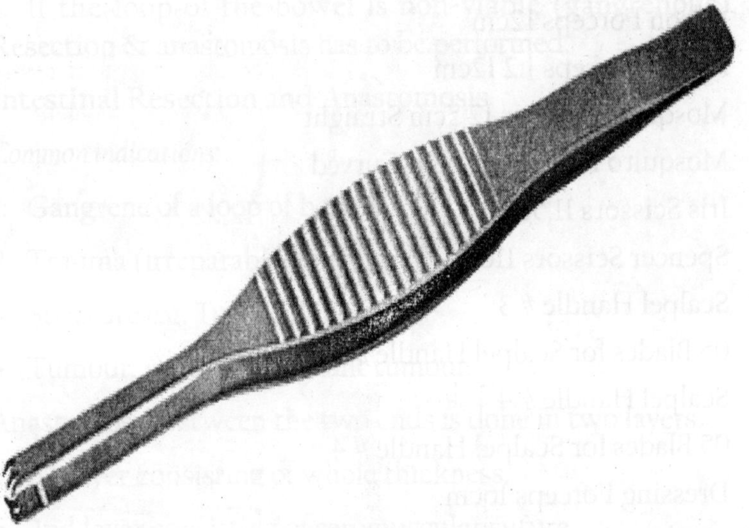

Fig. 0.2

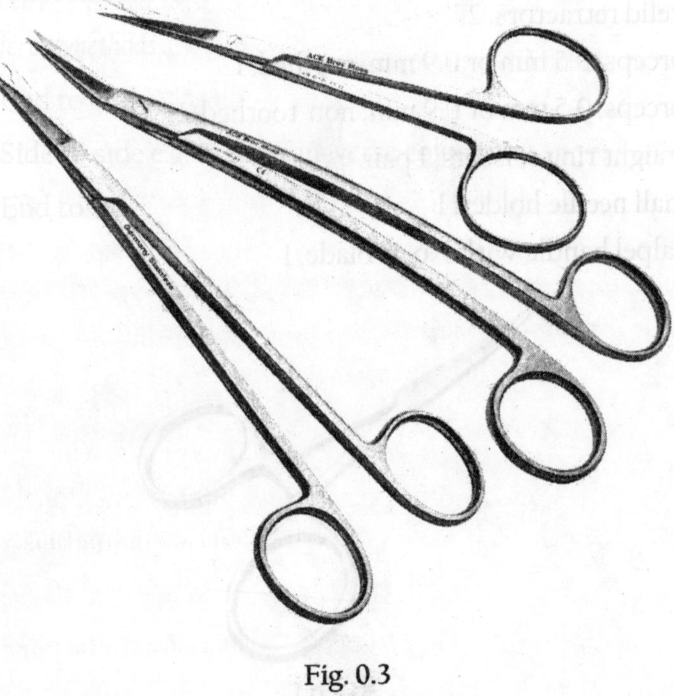

Fig. 0.3

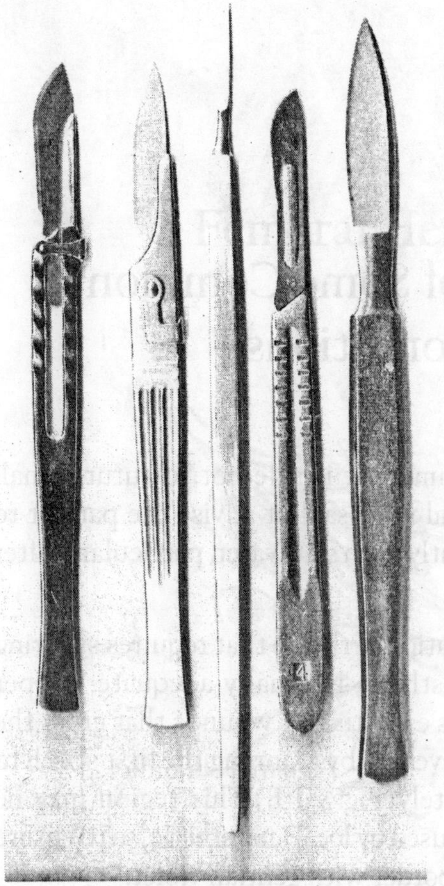

Fig. 0.4

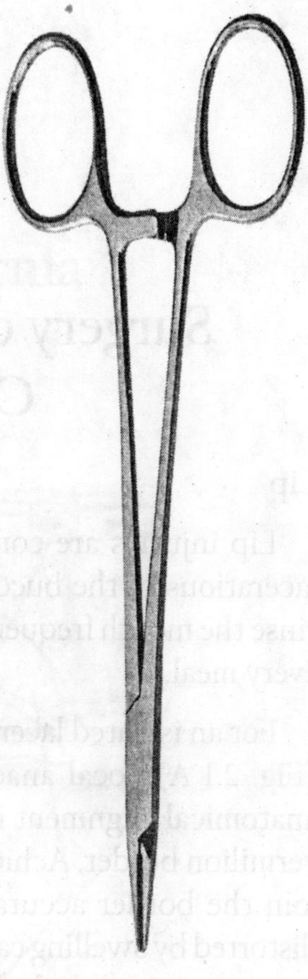

Fig. 0.5

3

Surgery of Some Common Conditions

Lip

Lip injuries are common. It is safe not to suture small lacerations of the buccal mucosa, but advise the patient to rinse the mouth frequently with salt water, particularly after every meal.

For an isolated laceration of the lip that requires suturing (Fig. 2.1 A), local anaesthesia is usually adequate. Proper anatomical alignment is essential for wounds that cross the vermilion border. Achieve this by planning the first stitch to join the border accurately(Fig. 2.1 B).This region may be distorted by swelling caused by local anaesthetic, so to ensure accuracy, premark the border with gentian violet.

After this key suture has been inserted, repair the rest of the wound in layers, starting with the mucosa and progressing to the muscles and finally the skin (Fig. 2.1 C, D, E). Use fine, interrupted sutures of 4/0 or 3/0 chromic catgut for the inner layers and thread or monofilament nylon for the skin.

Tongue

Most wounds of the tongue require no suturing and heal rapidly, but you may need to suture lacerations with a raised flap in either the lateral border or the dorsum of the tongue

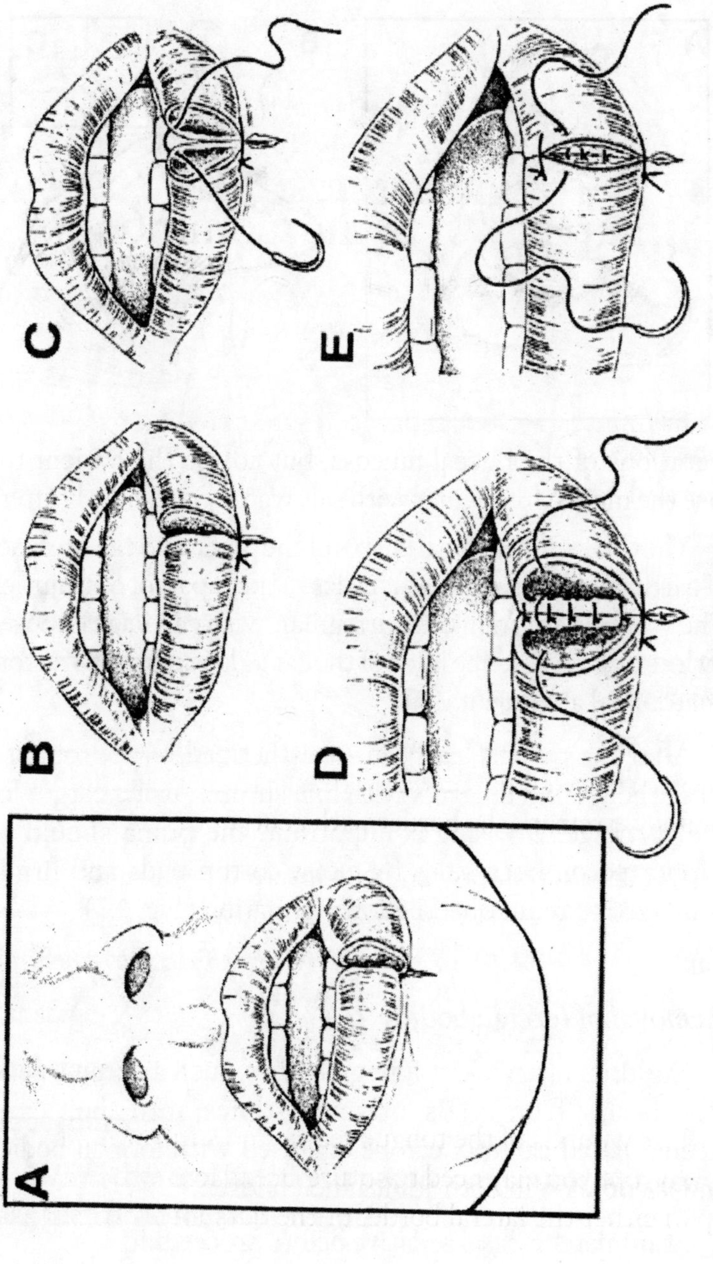

Fig. 2.1 A-E

(Fig. 2.2). Suture the flap to its bed with 4/0 or 3/0 buried, catgut stitches. Local anaesthesia is usually sufficient.

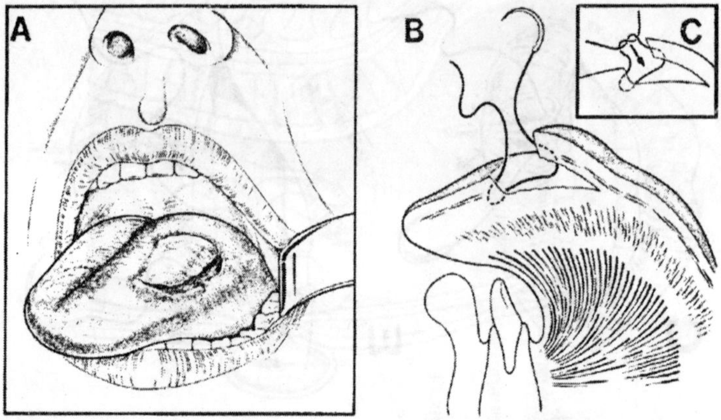

Ear and Nose

The three-dimensional curves of the pinna and the presence of cartilage can present difficulties in the repair of ear injuries. The wounds are commonly irregular, with cartilage exposed by loss of skin. Use the folds of the ear as landmarks to restore anatomical alignment.

After the patient has been anaesthetized, as appropriate, close the wound in layers with fine sutures, using catgut for the cartilage. Dressing is important: the pinna should be supported on both sides by moist cotton pads and firmly bandaged to reduce haematoma formation (Fig. 2.3).

Ear

Removal of foreign bodies

Children often insert foreign bodies, such as beans, peas, rice, beads, fruit seeds, or small stones, into their ears. Accumulated ear wax can be confused with foreign bodies and is common in both adults and children.

Administer a basal sedative before proceeding.

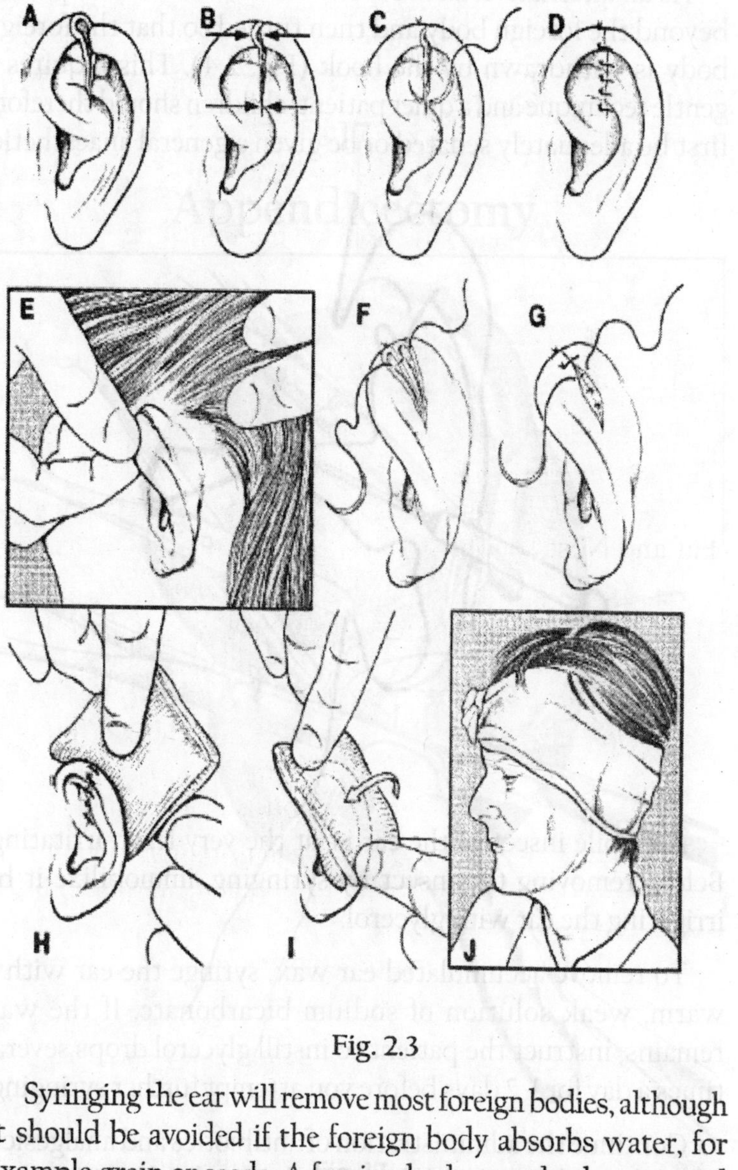

Fig. 2.3

Syringing the ear will remove most foreign bodies, although it should be avoided if the foreign body absorbs water, for example grain or seeds. A foreign body can also be removed by gentle suction through a soft rubber tube introduced into the ear to rest against the object. The procedure is simple, painless, and usually effective.

As an alternative, an aural curette or hook may be passed beyond the foreign body and then turned so that the foreign body is withdrawn by the hook (Fig. 2.4). This requires a gentle technique and a quiet patient; children should therefore first be adequately sedated or be given a general anaesthetic.

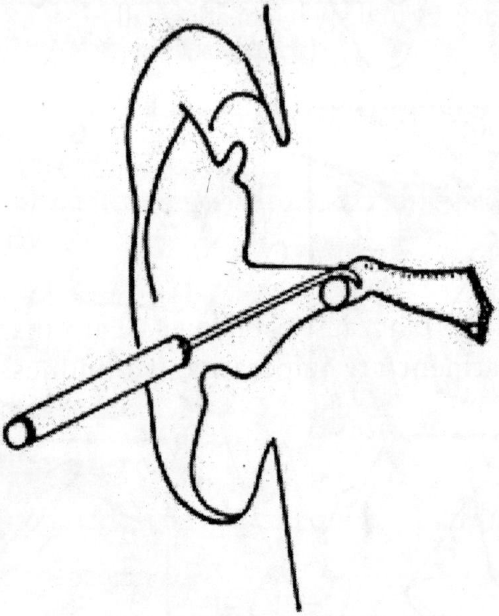

A mobile insect in the ear is, at the very least, irritating. Before removing the insect by syringing, immobilize it by irrigating the ear with glycerol.

To remove accumulated ear wax, syringe the ear with a warm, weak solution of sodium bicarbonate. If the wax remains, instruct the patient to instill glycerol drops several times a day for 1-2 days before you attempt further syringing.

Continue the administration of antibiotics and analgesics. Keep the auditory canal dry, and change the dressing when necessary.

Cellulitis of the Face

It may be a complication of facial wounds, carries the serious risk of cavernous-sinus thrombosis, so the patient's initial response to treatment with antibiotics. The organisms responsible are likely to be penicillin-sensitive. The patient must resist squeezing or otherwise manipulating any infected foci on the face, even if such foci ate small.

Eye

The purpose of eye surgery at the district hospital is to save sight and to prevent the progression of eye conditions that could produce further damage if left untreated. The surgical correction of squints and the treatment of congenital cataract should not be attempted. Eye injuries are common and are an important cause of blindness. Early diagnosis and proper treatment are imperative if blindness is to be prevented. Superficial injuries of the eyelid, conjunctiva, or cornea do not require surgical intervention. Providing that no foreign body is present, copiously irrigate the eyelid and eye with sterile physiological saline and apply tetracycline 1% eye ointment. Dress the eyelid and eye with a simple sterile eye pad, with the eyelids closed. Leave the dressing in place for 24 hours, and then re-examine the eye and eyelids. If the injury has resolved or is improving, continue applying tetracycline 1% eye ointment three times daily for 3 days. Otherwise inject gentamicin subcutaneously and arrange to refer the patient.

Small foreign bodies may be embedded superficially in the conjunctiva or cornea. If a foreign body is embedded in the conjunctiva, wash it out with sterile saline or, after administering a topical anaesthetic, wipe it away with a sterile, cotton- tipped applicator. Eversion of the lid may be necessary to expose the foreign body. If you suspect a corneal foreign body, first instill two drops of 2% sodium fluorescein to make the foreign body (or breach of the epithelium) easier to detect. Remove a superficial corneal foreign body with an eye spud or a 27-gauge needle, and then manage the eye as for a superficial injury.

Repairing a laceration of the eyelid. Laceration(A); inserting the key suture to align the lid margin (B); suturing the conjunctiva and tarsus (C, the knots arc tied away from the eyeball); suturing the skin and muscle (D).

Refer to hospital any patient with inflammation of the globe with hyphaema (blood in the anterior chamber). Place the patient at complete rest, with sedation if required, and patch both eyes. If intraocular pressure is elevated, as indicated by a total hyphaema or pain, administer acetazolamide 250 mg orally every 6 hours. Examine and dress the eye daily. If the hyphaema has not dearly improved in 5 days, refer the patient.

Lacerations and Penetrating Injuries

The patient should be anaesthetized as appropriate.

Eyelids

Make every attempt to preserve tissue, but carry out wound toilet and, if necessary, debridement. Do not shave the brow or invert hair-bearing skin into the wound. If the laceration involves the eyelid margin, place an intermarginal suture behind the eyelashes; precise alignment of the wound margins is essential (Fig. 3.1 A, B). Carry out the repair in two layers: the conjunctiva and tarsus with 6/0 catgut, and the skin and muscle (orbicularis oculi) with 6/0 thread (Fig. 3.1 C, D). Tie suture knots away from the eyeball.

Lacerations involving the inferior lacrimal canaliculus require canalicular repair, so the patient should be referred for specialized surgical management. If this is impossible, repair the lid margin and laceration as described above.

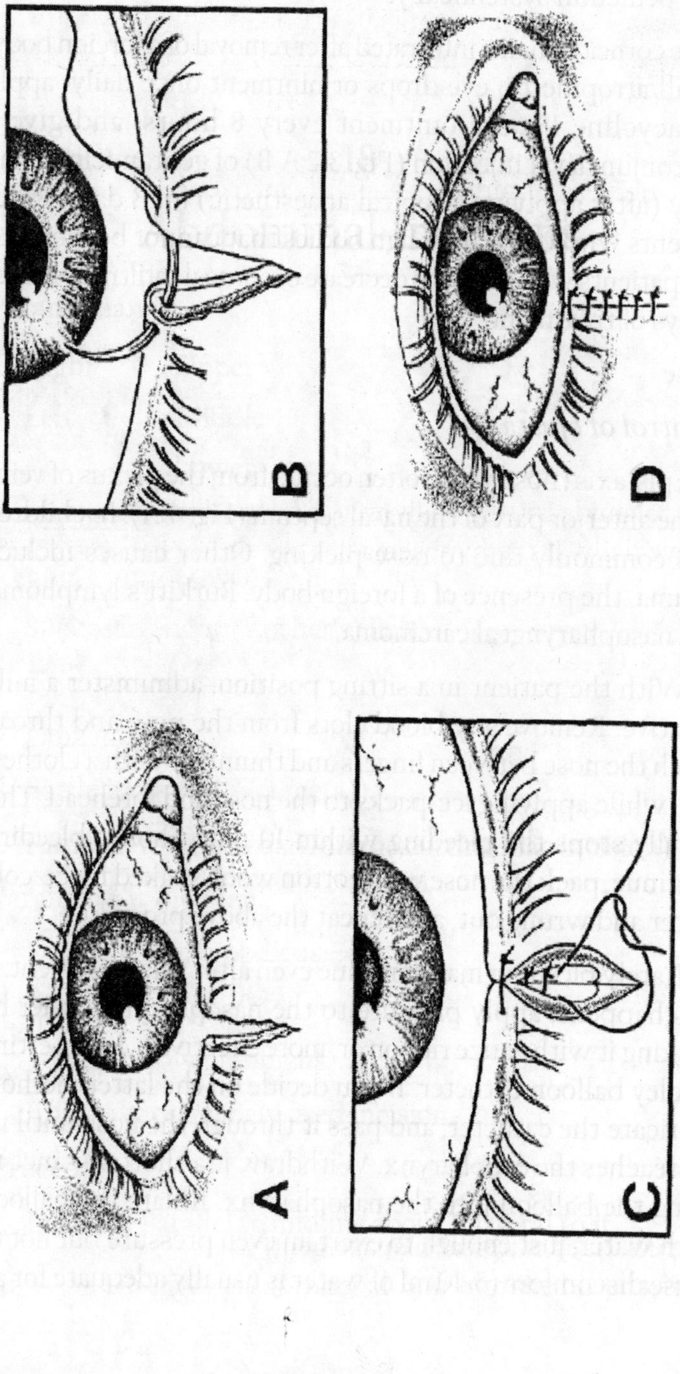

Fig. 3.1 (A-D)

Immunize the patient against tetanus with tetanus toxoid and give penicillin systemically.

If the cornea remains infiltrated after removal of a foreign body, instill atropine 1% eye drops or ointment once daily, apply tetracycline 1% eye ointment every 8 hours, and give a subconjunctival injection (Fig. 3.2 A B) of gentamicin 20 mg daily (after applying a topical anaesthetic) for 3 days. Refer patients with corneal foreign bodies that cannot be removed and patients who show no decrease of corneal infiltration after 3 days of treatment.

Nose

Control of epistaxis

Epistaxis (nosebleed) often occurs from the plexus of veins in the anterior part of the nasal septum (Fig. 4 A). In children it is commonly due to nose-picking. Other causes include trauma, the presence of a foreign body, Burkitt's lymphoma, and nasopharyngeal carcinoma.

With the patient in a sitting position, administer a mild sedative. Remove any blood clots from the nose and throat. Pinch the nose between fingers and thumb or with a clothes-peg, while applying ice-packs to the nose and forehead. This usually stops the bleeding within 10 min. Should bleeding continue, pack the nose with cotton wool, soaked in ice-cold water and wrung out, and repeat the above procedure.

Rarely bleeding may continue even after this treatment. If this happens, apply pressure to the nasopharynx either by packing it with gauze ribbon or, more effectively, by inserting a Foley balloon catheter. If you decide on the latter method, lubricate the catheter, and pass it through the nose until its tip reaches the oropharynx. Withdraw it a short distance to bring the balloon into the nasopharynx. Inflate the balloon with water, just enough to exert an even pressure but not to cause discomfort (5-10 ml of water is usually adequate for an

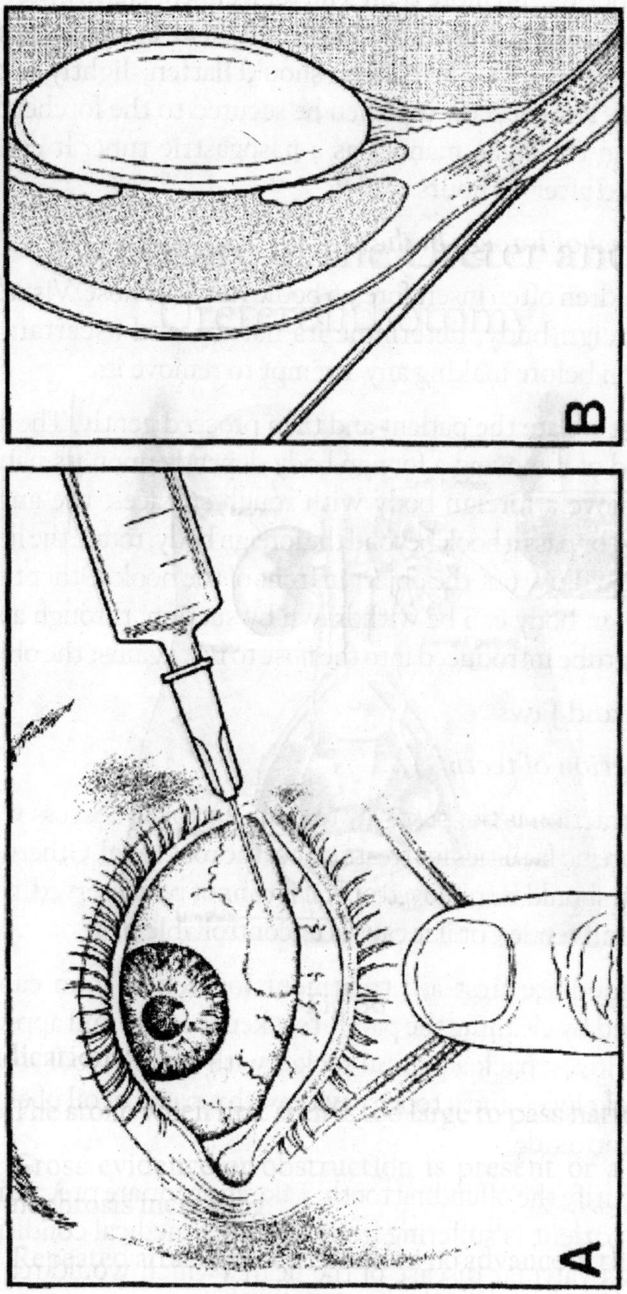

Fig. 3.2 (A-B)

adult, but use no more than 5 ml for a child). Gently pull the catheter forward until the balloon is held in the posterior choana (Fig. 4 B). The balloon should flatten slightly as this is done. The catheter can then be secured to the forehead or cheek in the same manner as a nasogastric tube. It can be removed after 48 hours.

Removal of foreign bodies

Children often insert foreign bodies into the nose. Visualize the foreign body, determine its nature, and ascertain its position before making any attempt to remove it.

First sedate the patient and then proceed gently. The best method of removing a foreign body depends upon its nature. To remove a foreign body with rough surfaces, use angled forceps, or pass a hook beyond the foreign body, rotate the hook, and then draw out the object in front of the hook. Other types of foreign body can be withdrawn by suction, through a soft rubber tube introduced into the nose to rest against the object.

Teeth and Jaws

Extraction of teeth

Extraction is the best way to drain an apical abscess when there are no facilities for treatment of the root canal. Otherwise, a tooth should be removed only if it cannot be preserved, if it is loose and tender, or if it causes uncontrollable pain.

Immediate first-aid treatment for dental pain can be afforded by cleaning the painful socket or cavity and applying oil of cloves; pack a painful socket with cotton wool soaked in oil of cloves and a tooth cavity with a paste of oil of cloves and zinc oxide.

Identify the offending tooth. Take appropriate precautions if the patient is suffering from any other medical conditions such as valvular disease of the heart (which would require prophylactic antibiotic cover), bleeding disorders, or diabetes.

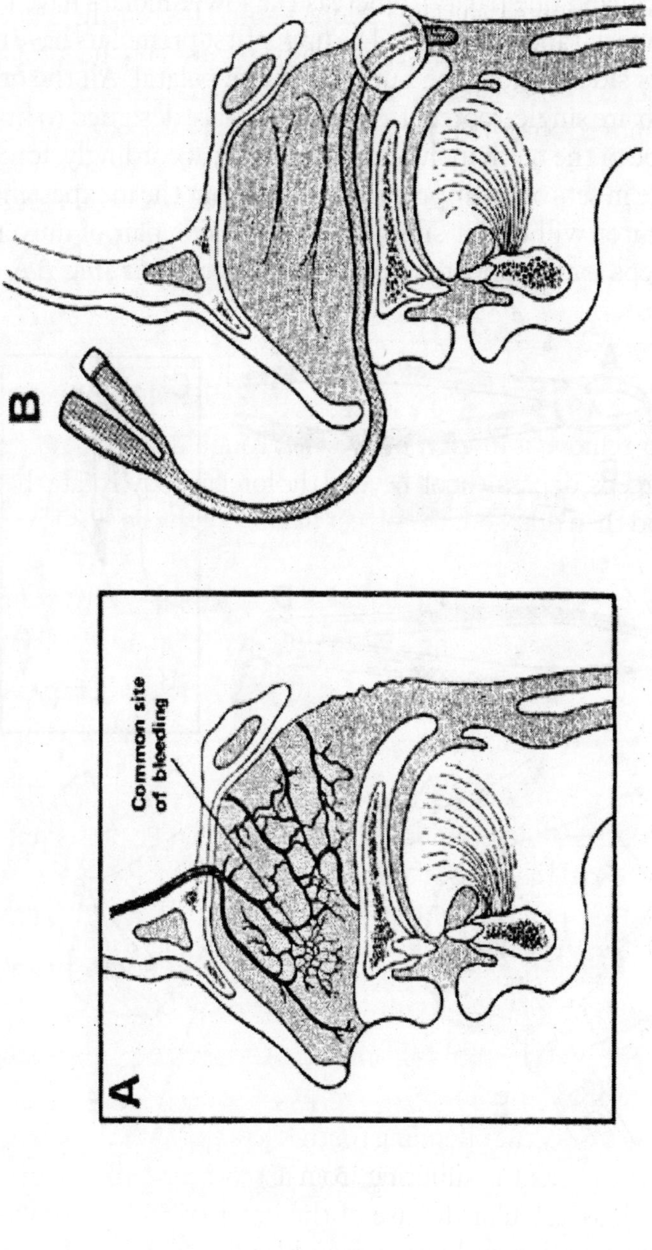

Fig. 4 (A-B)

It may be helpful to obtain a radiograph of the jaw. Check the patient's haemoglobin level and test the urine for sugar.

Remember that the upper molars have three roots, two buccal and one palatal, whereas the lower molars have two, one mesial and one distal. The upper first premolars have two roots side by side, one buccal and one palatal. All the other teeth are single-rooted. Dental forceps are designed to fit the shape of the teeth including their roots; accordingly, forceps come in sets of six appropriate shapes, but the inexperienced operator will find it simpler to rely on one pair of universal forceps for the upper jaw and one for the lower (Fig. 5 A-D).

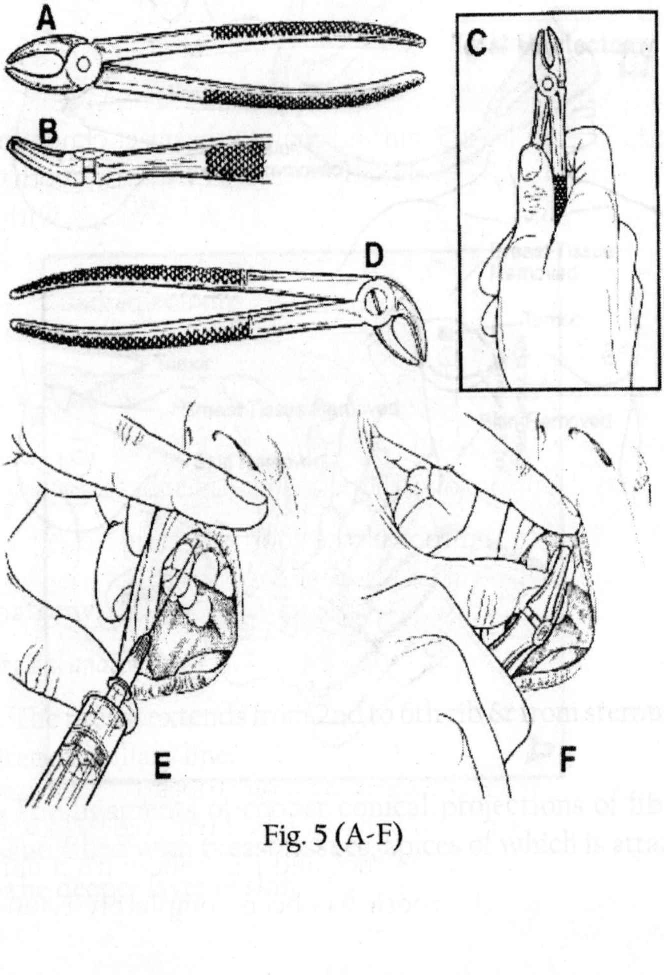

Fig. 5 (A-F)

Local infiltration analgesia should usually be sufficient for extraction of all but the lower molars, which may require a mandibular nerve block. Occasionally general anaesthesia may be appropriate.

Administer a sedative to children and anxious adults. Seat the patient in a chair with a back high enough to support the head. After the patient has rinsed the mouth, swab the gum with 70% ethanol. To effect local infiltration anaesthesia, insert a 25-gauge, 25 mm needle at the junction of the mucoperiosteum of the gum and the cheek, parallel to the axis of the tooth (Fig. 5 E). Advance the needle 0.5 to 1 cm, level with the apex of the tooth, just above the periosteum. The bevel of the needle should face the tooth. Infiltrate the tissues with 1 ml of lidocaine and epinephrine and repeat the procedure on the other side of the tooth. Wait at least 5 min and confirm the onset of numbness before handling the tooth. Separate the gum from the tooth with a straight elevator. While supporting the alveolus with the thumb and finger of your other hand, apply the forceps to either side of the crown, parallel with the long axisof the root. Position the palatal or lingual blade first. Push the blades of the forceps up or down the periodontal membrane on either side of the tooth, depending on which jaw you are working on (Fig. 5 F). The secret of successful extraction is to drive the blades of the forceps as far up or down the periodontal membrane as possible.

Firmly grip the root of the tooth with the forceps and loosen the tooth with gentle rocking movements from buccal to lingual Drpalatal side. If the tooth does not begin to move, loosen the forceps, push them deeper, and repeat the rocking movements. Avoid excessive lateral force on a tooth, as this can lead to its fracture.

Carefully inspect the extracted tooth to confirm its complete removal. A broken root is best removed by loosening the tissue between the root and the bone with a curved elevator. After the tooth has been completely removed, squeeze the sides of the socket together for a minute or two and place a dental roll over the socket. Instruct the patient to bite on it for a short while.

After the patient has rinsed the mouth, inspect the cavity for bleeding. Repair lacerations and arrest profuse bleeding that will not stop, even when pressure is applied, with mattress sutures of 0 catgut across the cavity. Warn the patient not to rinse the mouth again for the first 24 hours or the blood clot may be washed out, leaving a dry socket (with the risk of alveolar osteitis). The patient should rinse the mouth frequently with saline during the next few days.

A simple analgesic may be needed when the effects of the local anaesthetic have worn off. It is worth warning the patient against exploring the cavity with a finger, explaining that the numbness is temporary and will last only for an hour or so. Haemorrhage after dental extraction is a common emergency and can usually be controlled by simple pressure over the socket or, if necessary, by suturing the gum. Haemostatic substances have little advantage over simple pressure. If gross dental sepsis occurs, administer penicillin for 48 hours and consider giving tetanus toxoid, if necessary.

Fractures of the jaw

Fractures of the maxilla require specialist care, but mandibular fractures can often be treated in the district hospitaL Fractures of the ramus and the condyle of the mandible are usuallyclosed and require little reduction. Fractures of the body of the mandible are usually compound, through the alveolar margin, and necessitate immobilization, which can be achieved by direct wiring between the teeth on either side of the fracture or by interdental wiring between the two jaws (when the upper jaw is stable).

Diagnosis and treatment

If the patient presents with a suspected mandibular fracture, note any altered dental occlusion and, if necessary, confirm the fracture by X-ray examination. Check for other injuries, and decide on the priorities for treatment. Keeping the airway clear is most important; the patient should therefore be nursed lying on the side or in a sitting position with the head well forward. Give penicillin and tetanus toxoid.

With the maintenance of a clear airway and the administration of antibiotics, the patient's condition can be expected to improve considerably in the first 24 hours.

The only urgent indication for wiring a mandibular fracture is instability of a comminuted fracture through the incisors. In this instance, the tongue may need to be held forward temporarily by a stitch through its tip and the teeth wired immediately. Otherwise wiring can be delayed until the patient's condition is stable.

Interdental wiring of the jaws

Technique

After sedating the patient, you may gently insert interdental eyelets without anaesthesia, but nerve block (of the inferior alveolar nerve) and infiltration anaesthesia are much preferred. General anaesthesia is an alternative but, should the patient present with an airway that is difficult to manage or with a full stomach, it will be extremely hazardous if the anaesthetist is inexperienced.

Clean the patient's mouth. Examine the jaws for any obvious wounds, which should be sutured. Locate the fracture (Fig. 6 A) and reduce it as far as possible. If there is any doubt about the viability of a tooth in the fracture line, remove it. The method of wiring the jaw will depend on the state of the remaining teeth. Choose the nearest two healthy teeth, one on each side of the fracture line, and pass a 16 em length of wire (twisted to make an eyelet on the buccal side) between them from the buccal to the lingual side (Fig. 6 B). Pass the ends back to surround the teeth, carrying one end through the eyelet and then tightening it by twisting it against its fellow (Fig. 6 C-E). Cut the excess wire short and bend it away from the lip to lie flush along the jaw. Repeat the procedure on a matching pair of teeth in the upper jaw (Fig. 6 F). Fix the mandible to the maxilla by wiring the upper and lower eyelets together immediately or, if there are any worries about the patient's airway at the end of anaesthesia, at a later session (Fig. 6 G). Additional teeth may be wired together if necessary.

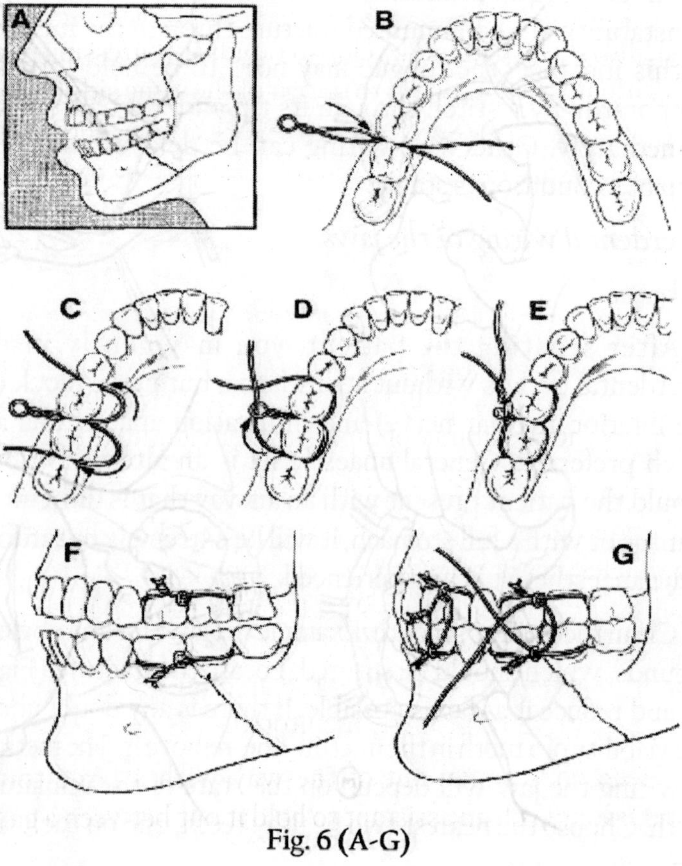

Fig. 6 (A-G)

The jaw should be kept immobilized until the fracture unites: 6 weeks for an adult but only 3-4 weeks for a child. During this time, the patient should continue to brush the teeth regularly, except perhaps for the first few days when the mouth can be gently syringed. The patient's diet must, of course, be fluid or semi-solid.

Throat

Non-emergency operations on the throat (in particular tonsillectomy) should not be attempted at the private clinics or small hospitals.

Incision and drainage of peritonsillar abscess:

Peritonsillar abscess (quinsy) is a complication of acute tonsillitis. The patient develops a rapidly progressing pain in the throat which radiates to the ear of the same side and soon becomes unbearable. The neck is held rigid, and there is associated fever, dysarthria, dysphagia, drooling of saliva, trismus, and foul breath. Clinical examination will confirm fever and will usually reveal cervical lymphadenopathy on the side of the lesion. Local swelling causes the anterior tonsillar pillar to bulge and displaces the soft palate and uvula towards the opposite side. The overlying mucosa is inflamed, sometimes with a small spot already discharging pus. Keep in mind the possibility of diphtheria or glandular fever.

Administer a basal sedative and place the patient in a sitting position with the head supported. Surface anaesthesia is preferable and will avoid the risk of inhalation of the abscess contents, which can occur under general anaesthesia. Spray the region of the abscess with 2-4% lidocaine. Never use ethyl chloride for this purpose, as the amount absorbed by the patient cannot be properly monitored.

Keep the tongue out of the way with a large tongue depressor or ask an assistant to hold it out between a gauze-covered finger and thumb as you proceed. Perform a preliminary needle aspiration (Fig. 7 A), and then incise the most prominent part of the swelling near the anterior pillar (Fig. 7 B). Introduce the point of a pair of artery forceps or sinus forceps into the incision, and open the jaws of the forceps to improve drainage (Fig. 7 C). Provide suction, if necessary.

Instruct the patient to gargle with warm salt water several times a day for about 5 days. Continue the administration of antibiotics for 7-10 days and analgesics for as long as necessary.

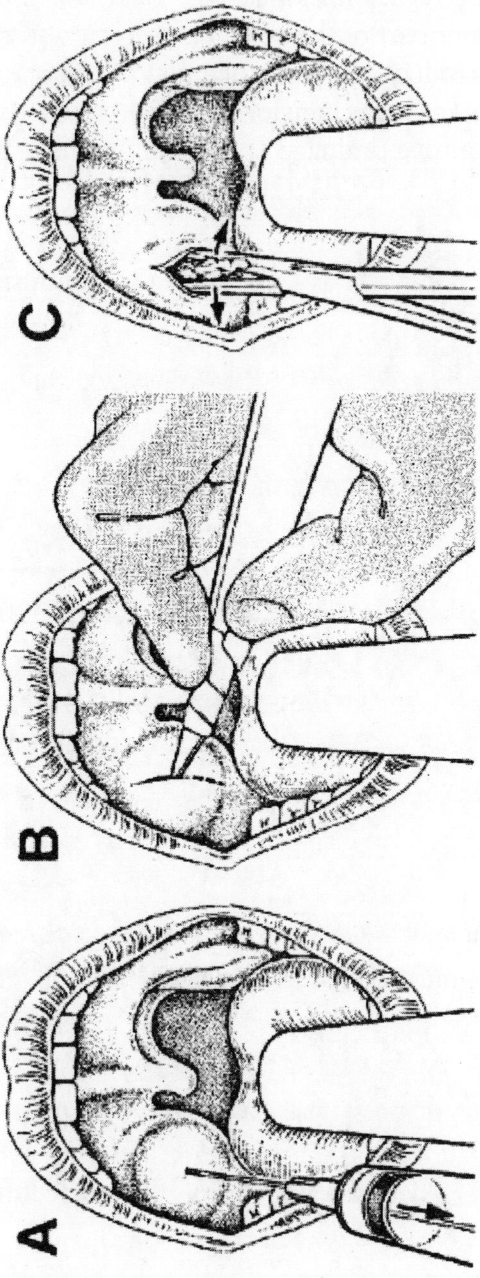

Fig. 7 (A-C)

33

Tracheostomy

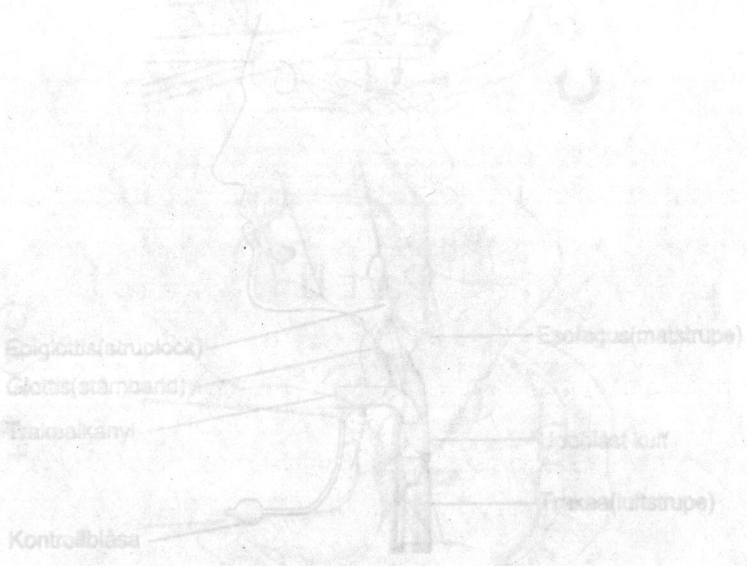

Fig. 33

Indications:

A. To relieve acute respiratory obstruction

1. Laryngeal diphtheria
2. Impaction of a foreign body
3. Oedema of the glottis
4. Bilateral recurrent nerve injury at thyroidectomy

Part II
Operative Surgery

1

Sterilisation

Definitions:

Sterilisation is a process whereby all living organisms including spores are destroyed whereas disinfection is a process which destroys only the vegetative forms of organisms but does not kill the spores.

Antiseptic surgery aims at killing the micro-organisms present in the wound by .the use of antiseptics like germicides, etc.

Aseptic surgery (Asepsis) is the technique employed i.e. sterilisation of all articles coming into contact with the patient, whereby micro-organisms are prevented from gaining access to uninfected tissues.

Blunt Instruments

These are sterilised by either of the following methods

1. Boiling in boiling water for at least 45 minutes.
2. Autoclaving (Steaming under pressure).

   Usually a heat of 120 degree celcius with 15 lb pressure for 30 minutes.
3. Formalin vapour steriliser : This useful apparatus is also used for sterilisation of all instruments.
4. When an instrument is very urgently required to be sterilised, it may be exposed to direct heat i.e, flaming.

Sharp Instruments:

These are sterilised with chemicals. Commonly used chemicals are:

a. *Lysol:* Sharp instruments (scissors, blades, needles etc.) are usually put in concentrated lysol for atleast half an hour. Before use, after taking out of lysol solution with Lifter, the instrument must be thoroughly rinsed with sterile water.

b. *Cidex (2% glutaraldehyde):* Instruments (even blunt instruments, endoscopes etc.) can be put in activated solution for sterilisation. Time required for destruction of pathogenic spores is 4 to 10 hours. Time required for distinction is only 15 minutes.

Linen:

Draping sheets, gowns, gloves, etc. are sterilised by autoclaving.

Catheters:

Rubber drains, rubber tubes are sterilised by boiling or autoclaving for 10 minutes.

2
Suture Materials

An ideal suture should be strong but slender, flexible to apply & comfortable. It should be smooth on surface so that it offers no cavities for bacterial growth. It should be non-reactive & have good knotting security.

Absorbable Sutures

1. *Natural: Catgut*

It is from the submucosa of sheep intestines. (The word catgut has possibly come from kit gut which means the string of the violin).

Processing & Sterilisation:

a. The submucous coat of the sheep intestines is washed with ether to dissolve fat.
b. Then it is immersed in carbolic acid for 8 days so that the spore bearing organisms are destroyed.
c. It is supplied in airtight packs containing 70% alcohol (as preservative) & 5% glycerine (which keeps it soft).

Plain catgut: It is absorbed in the tissues within a week.

Chromic catgut:

It is obtained by processing the catgut in salts of chromic acid for a variable period. Chromic or chromicised catgut remains in the tissues for 10 to 40 days.

As time passes catgut is absorbed by enzymatic digestion.

The size of the catgut is according to its thickness (e.g. 4/0, 3/0, 2/0, 1/0, 1.2).

Advantages:

The advantage of catgut is that it is absorbed in the tissues therefore can be used even in the presence of infection.

Disadvantages:

a. It is a foreign protein & may cause tissue irritation, necrosis & infection (stitch abscess, catgut sinus).

b. The tensile strength diminishes after 3-4 days.

2. Synthetic:

a. Dexon (homopolymer of glycolide)

b. Vicryl (copolymer of glycolide & lactide)

c. P.D.S. (homopolymer of polydioxanone).

They have prolonged absorption time (more than 90 days) and cause minimal tissue reaction but knotting qualities are less satisfactory .

Non Absorable Sutures

E.g. Thread (cotton or linen), silk, polyester, polyamide, polypropylene, polyethylene, steel. They may be in the shape of monofilament, multifilament, braided or twisted.

Thread, silk, etc. can be sterilised by boiling or autoclaving. Commonly used non-absorbable suture materials are thread, silk (for skin suture, ligation of blood vessels etc.) & prolene.

Prolene (Monofilament polpropylene): is used for Hernia repair, suturing of sheath, tendon etc. Steel wire is used for suturing (fixation) fractured bony ends e.g. patella, olecranon, sternum, and also in dental surgery (Inter dental wiring for fracture mandible).

3
Nomenclature of Operations

1. The sufflx "Ostomy" denotes making an opening into a hollow organ or cavity & closing it after dealing the pathology e.g. laparotomy, gastrotomy.
2. The suffix "Ostomy" denotes making an opening into a cavity & maintaining it to the exterior e.g. colostomy, tracheostomy.
3. The sufflx "Ectomy" denotes excision or removal of some structure e.g. cholecystectomy, orchidectomy.
4. The suffix "Lysis" denotes mobilization of an organ e.g, neurolysis.
5. The suffix "Pexy" denotes fixation of the organ in its normal anatomical position e.g. orchidopexy.
6. The suffix "Plasty" denotes plastic operations for reforming a structure e.g. pyloroplasty, urethroplasty.

4

Planning for Operation

Operation may be

1. Elective surgery: i.e. planned procedure e.g. cholecystec-tomy, hernioplasty.
2. Emergency surgery: where urgent intervention is required, e.g. strangulated hernia, perforated peptic ulcer.

In any Operation:

1. Pre-operative assessment and preparation: Routine investigation e.g. haemogram, urinalysis, correct anaemia, treat chest infection or any septic focus, control diabetes if present.
2. Shaving and antiseptic dressing in the ward.
3. Choice of anaesthesia & Premedication–

I. General

II. Local

General	Local
Atropine (0.65 mg) or Glycopyrolate	Pethidine (100 mg)
Phenergan (50 mg)	Phenergen
Diazepam	Diazepam Pentazocine

4. Position of the patient: Supine

   Lateral

   Kidney position

   Lithotomy position for perineal surgery.

- For Neck surgery sand bag between the shoulder blades.

5. Skin preparation: Savlon (Cetrimide & Chlorhexidine) Tincture iodine, Bovtdone iodine.
6. Towelling.
7. Skin incision.
8. Procedure and findings.
9. Drainage tube, if required: Tube drain

   Corrugated drain

   Suction drain (Redivae or portavac).
10. Closure.

II. Post-operative management.

5

Anaesthesia

1. General Anaesthesia

Reversible loss of conciousness and sensations with muscle relaxation and abolition of reflexes.

I. Types:

i. Spontaneous: The patient breathes himself.

Drugs used are :

a. Halothane

b. Ether

c. Trichloroethylene.

ii. Controlled: The anaesthetist ventilates patient after using the muscle relaxants.

Oxygen and Nttrous Oxide are used alongwith other agents (drugs).

a. Depolarising, b. Non-depolarising.

2. Pre-Operative Evaluation:

a. Routine investigations: Haemogram, Blood Sugar, X-Ray etc.

E.C.G. for patients above 35 years.

Renal function and Liver function tests in selected cases.

b. Specific medication

Control of diabetes (by insulin), hypertension and chest infection.

Correction of anaemia.

History of taking medications.

3. Over-Night (or 6 to 8 hours) fasting prior to surgery as

a. Protective reflexes are abolished under General anaesthesia.

b. To prevent regurgitation: Aspiration.

4. Pre-Anaesthetic Medication:

a. Sedatives to allay anxiety of the patient e.g. Diazepam, Nitrazepam etc.

b. Anti-Cholinergic drugs:

i. Atropine, 0.6 mg. I.M. given 30 to 40 minutes before surgery.

Or

ii. Glycopyrrolate (Atropine substitute), 0.02 mg./kg.

Advantages:

a. Tachycardia much less.

b. C.N.S. toxicity absent.

c. Analgesics and Sedatives e.g. Pentazocine 0.5 rug/kg. I.M. or Diazepam.

d. Broncho dilators and Corticoid, if indicated.

5. Induction Agents:

a. Sodium-pentothal (Ultra short acting barbiturate) Dose I.V.-4 mg./kg.

b. Methohexitone (methylated thiobarb)

Dose LV.- 1 mg./kg.

c. Ketamine hydrochloride

Duration of action

LV.-15 minutes

LM.-30 minutes.

Causes dissociative anaesthesia: higher centres are dissociated from reticular activating system.

Dose: Induction- o.5-2 mg/kg. LV.

4-6 mg./kg. LM.

Advantages:

i. Good analgesia.

ii. Total amnesia and catalepsy.

Disadvantnges:

i. Severe hallucinations.

ii. Increases heart rate and Blood Pressure.

Contra indications:

i. Increased intra-cranial pressure.

ii. Ischaemic heart disease.

iii. Psychiatric patients.

d. Diazepam, Phenergan, Fentanyl, Droperidol etc. are sometimes used.

6. Method of Induction and Intubation

(Common to both Procedures-Spontaneous & Controlled)

i. LV. drip.

ii. Check pulse. B.P. and air entry.

iii. Pulse Oxymeter and E.C.G. selected cases.

Leads are placed in position in

iv. Sodium pentothal is given slowly I.V. while monitoring the pulse.

End point checked by eyelash/eyelid reflexes.

v. Scoline 1.5-2 mg./kg. I.V. given

vi. Continue oxygenation.

vii. Intermittent positive pressure respiration with a reservoir bag-till total paralysis is evident (Patient cannot breathe himself). l.

viii. Endo-tracheal intubation is done with the help of Laryngo-scope.

ix. ETT is connected to Maggil's circuit (Boyl's machine).

x. After 2-3 blasts of 100% Oxygen, Nitrous oxide (N2O) is started, ratio being 60 : 40.

xi. Air way is passed.

7. *Spontaneous Anaesthesia:*

i. Start halothane/ether through the Boyl's machine/ Vaporisers after the above mentioned induction and intubation.

ii. Once the patient starts breathing, stop _ventillating (effect of scoline, the short acting relaxant, passes off within few minutes).

iii. Maintain the level of anaesthesia.

iv. At the end of the operation

a. stop anaesthetic agent.

b. do an oral suction.

c. wait for the return of pharyngeal reflexes. (d) remove endo-tracheal tube

8. Controlled Anaesthesia:

Non-depolarising, long acting muscle relaxants e.g. gallamine or pancuronium etc. are used to paralyse the patient. Ventillation is continued throughout with O_2 and NO_2.

Neostigmine I.V. is given at the end of the operation for the reversal of the effects of relaxant.

Ventillation is continued till spontaneous respiration sets in.

Endotracheal tube is removed after oral suction and return of reflexes.

Chock muscle power by protrusion of tongue.

9. Complications

a. Aspiration (Mandelson's Syndrome)

   Chemical pneumonitis.

   H_2 antagonist antacids etc. may be given as preventive measure.

b. Cardiac arrest: Because of anaesthetic agents like Pentothal or hypotension and hypoxia.

c. Post recovery: nausea, vomiting and aspiration, hypotension.

d. Intubation : trauma to vocal cords.

e. I. V. line : haematoma, thrombophlebitis, air embolism.

f. Pulmonary: bronchospasm, chest infection.

2. Local Anaesthesia

l. Definition:

Temporary loss of sensation and relief of pain due to depression of nerve conduction beyond the point of application in a restricted area of body.

2. *Methods:*

   Surface anaesthesia (topical).

   Infiltration anaesthesia.

   Field block.

   Nerve block.

   Spinal anaesthesia.

   Epidural anaesthesia.

3. *Principles:*

a. Proper knowledge of the regional anatomy.

b. Proper local anaesthetic agent:

   i. Sufficient concentration.

   ii. Duration of surgery (1 to 2 hrs.)

c. Patient's wish.

d. Contraindications and history of allergy.

e. Resuscitation measures ready.

4. *Drug:*

A. Xylocaine (Lignocaine) Concentration

   Infiltration 0.5 to 1%

   Nerve block 2%

   Jelly Ointment 5%

   Topical 4%

B. Bupivacaine (Sensorcaine)

   Concentration : 0.25 to 1%

   For local blocks, infiltration & sustained action.

5. *Dose:*

Xylocaine (a) Without adrenaline = 3 - 5 mg/kg

(b) With adrenaline = 5 - 7 mg/kg

Duration (a) Without adrenaline

(b) With adrenaline = 45 mins to 1 hour. = 1 - 1.5 hours.

Sensorcaine : Dose - 2 mg/Kg.

Note: Adrenaline (1 : 2,000) : causes Vasoconstriction, hence less oozing and delayed absorption.

Contraindicated in Hypertension & Myocardial infarction.

6. *Complications:*

Over dosage-Causes restlessness, vertigo. tremors

Convulsions, hypotension, cardiac failure and/or respiratory failure.

Management is done by:

a. I.V. diazepam/Pentothal.
b. Short acting muscle relaxants.
c. Ventillation.
d. I.V. fluid & Vasopressor drugs.

3. Spinal Anaesthesia

1. *Definition:*

A technique, which causes complete blockade of the anterior and posterior nerve roots and the autonomic ganglia, by the introduction of a local anaesthetic agent into the subarachnoid space through an intervertebral space.

2. *Indications:*

i. Surgery below the umbilicus, specially pelvic surgery, surgery on the lower limb, hernia repair, prostatectomy etc.

ii. Patients in whom general anaesthesia is contraindicated e.g. in C.O.P.D. patients.

3. *Contraindications:*

Septicaemia, shock, spinal cord lesions, Local skin infection & Bleeding disorders.

4. *Drug:* Xylocaine 5% (2 c.c.) or Bupivacaine.

5. *Technique:*

a. Position

i. Sitting on the edge of the operation table with complete flexion of the neck and trunk.

ii. Lateral: Lower limb flexed at the knee joint as far as possible with complete flexion of the neck and trunk.

b. Part is prepared and infiltrated with Xylocaine (0.5 to 1%).

A spinal needle is introduced into the L4-L5 intervertebral space and directed towards the umbilicus. Free flow of C.S.F. is checked after the loss of the first resistance. Adequate amount of the drug is injected.

6. *Complications:*

a. Immediate:

i. Hypotension: mainly due to sympathetic blockade.

Sympathetomimetic drug e.g. Mephentine is given intravenously.

ii. Cardio-respiratory failure (total spinal)

- Intubation ventillation & resuscitation are required. (iii) Vomiting.

b. Delayed:

i. Headache

ii. Backache

iii. Retention of urine

iv. Cauda equina syndrome.

4. Epidural Anaesthesia

1. Direct block of the spinal nerve roots in the epidural space.
2. *Technique:*

   a. Hanging drop technique-drop sucked inside due to negative pressure.

   b. Loss of resistance technique.
3. *Drug:* Lignocaine (1%)

   Bupivacaine (0.5%)
4. Indications and Contraindications same as that of spinal anaesthesia
5. Advantages over Spinal anaesthesia:

   Duration of action: more.

   Chances of C.S.F. contamination: absent.

   Hypotension : less severe.

   Headache: absent.
6. *Disadvantages:*

   Backache: more severe

   Anaesthesia- patchy : whereas in spinal

   It is uniform.

6

Postoperative Complications

Postoperative complications may be

1. *General:*

a. Respiratory Atelectasis

Pneumonia

Pulmonary embolism (following D.V.T.).

b. Cardiac	Myocardial infarction Deep
c. Thrombotic	Venous thrombosis Thrombophlebitis.
d. Urinary	
Retention of urine-	
	Tubular necrosis (renal failure, viz., anuria, oliguria).
	Urinary tract infection.
e. Dehydration	Because of third-space sequestration of fluids in the operative site.
f. Overhydration	In patients with impaired cardiac or renal function.

2. *Local:*

a. Haemorrhage

b. Wound infection

c. Wound disruption (dehiscence)

d. Other specific complications following the particular surgery.

Postoperative complications can also be grouped:

a. Immediate: within first 24 hours.

b. Early: up to 3 weeks postoperatively.

c. Late: during any subsequent period after patient has left the hospital.

Postoperative complications in Abdominal surgery:

I. General

II. Local

As mentioned above.

Haemorrhage:

Reactionary haemorrhage (within 6 to 24 hours).

Paralytic Ileus:

Wound infections. including intrabdominal abscesses.

Peritonitis:

Secondary haemorrhage (7-14 days after operation).

Wound disruption.

Anastomotic leak (if anastomosis has been done).

Intestinal obstruction (due to adhesions).

Incisional hernia.

Recurrence of the disease or symptoms.

7
Abscess Drainage

The treatment of abscess is incision and drainage. In case of doubt it is safer to put in a needle and confirm the presence of pus by aspiration.

Hilton's method of drainage of Abscess:

Incision in the skin and deep fascia over the most prominent part.

A sinus forceps is thrust into the abscess cavity and its blades are opened to enlarge the opening.

A drain is put inside or the cavity is packed. Dressing is changed on alternate days.

Parotid Abscess:

Vertical incision over the most prominent part. Cut skin and then incise the parotid fascia transversely to avoid injury to fascial nerve. Thrust in a sinus forceps. Put in a drain or pack.

Fluctuation may not be evident due to tense parotid fascia. If left untreated, it may burst open in the ear at the junction of bony and cartilagenous meatus.

Breast Abscess:

Radial incision to avoid injury to lactiferous ducts.

Thrust the sinus forceps.

Break all the loculi with finger.

Pack with gauze soaked in E.C.

See that the drainage is dependent.

Counter drainage. if the abscess is situated in upper quadrant.

Ischio Rectal Abscess:

Anaesthesia: General or Local (Pundendal block). Cruciate incision (+ shaped).

Excise overhanging skin so that the wound becomes diamond shaped.

Explore the cavity, break down any septa and remove the necrotic tissue.

Pack the wound with E.C. guaze. Dressing daily or alternate days.

Delay in opening ischio-rectal. abscess may result in fistula-in-ano.

8

Venesection (Cut Down)

Indications:

1 I. V. Infusion for longer periods.

2. In shocked patients (as in the case of a Burn).
3. I. V. alimentation (feeding).

Veins:

Antecubital fossa (basilic vein).

Medial malleolus : long saphenous vein.

Procedure:

Local anaesthesia.

tourniquet.

1. Transverse incision over the vein.
2. Cut skin, clear superficial fascia.
3. Isolate the vein.
4. Pass two ligatures around the vein.
5. Distal one is tied.
6. Proximal one is half tied and its ends are kept loose.
7. A nick is made in the vein between the ligatures with scissors.

8. Canula or polythene tube is introduced upwards.
9. Proximal ligature is tied to enclose it.
10. Skin is stitched.

Complications:

Thrombophlebitis

Thrombosis

Local infection.

9

Skin Grafting

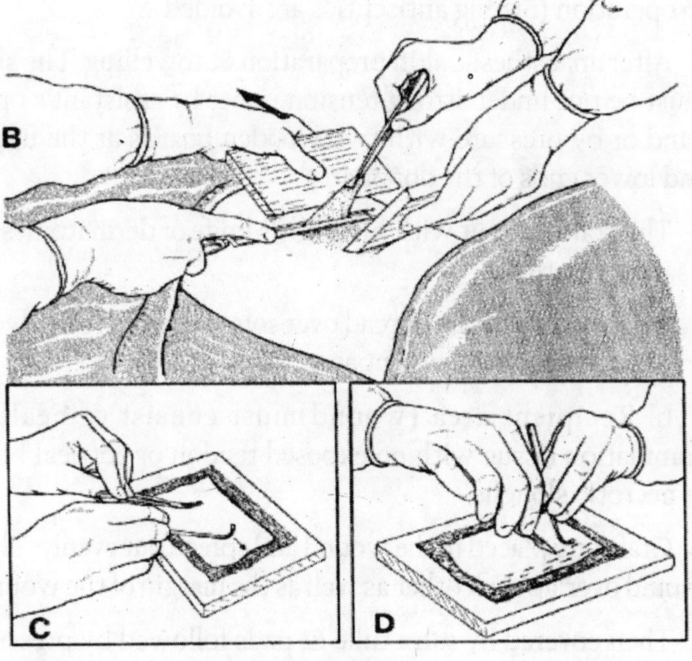

Fig. 9

Indications : Extensive raw wound as a result of

a. Deep burns
b. Trauma
c. Removal of malignant growth or callous ulcer.

Types of Skin Grafting:

A. Free Grafts:

1. Partial Thickness (Thiersch) Grafts (10 to 30 mu in thickness)

a. Preparation of donor site (usually the anterior surface of the thigh & forearm).

Shaving & cleaning with either soap or spirit, 24 hrs. prior to operation (Strong antiseptics are avoided).

After anaesthesia, skin preparation & towelling. The skin must be put under strong tension either by assistant's open hand or by pressure with two wooden boards at the upper and lower ends of the donor area.

The grafts are cut with a Humby's knife or dermatomes by a sawing motion.

Detached grafts are spread over sofra tulle & are ready for transplantation to recipient area.

b. Recipient area (wound)must consist of healthy granulation tissue with no exposed tendon or cortical bone or necrotic sloughs.

Grafts are placed in the wound and spread out evenly. They should overlap each other as well as the margin of the wound.

Then covered by safra tulle & pads followed by pressure bandage.

Dressing is changed after 7 to 8 days. It must be soaked with saline before removal from the wound.

2. Full Thickness (Wolfe)Grafts: These grafts are better than the thiersch grafts in that they have no tendency to contract and are of better colour and are ideal for the face or palm. The survival of the grafts depends on early vascularisation as opposed to partial thickness grafts which may live on exudate (lymph) for the time being.

3. Pinch or Reverdin Graft : These are small (1/4 inch) cones of skin consisting of whole thickness at the central part & epidermis at the periphery.

B. *Pedicle Graft:*

These grafts are suitable for the hand and foot and to repair deep defects in the face.

1. Rotational Flaps: The flap is made from the neighbourhood of the wound and is turned or rotated on their own blood supply to cover the defect.
2. Direct Pedicle Grafts : This method is applicable when the donor area can be brought into close proximity with the reciptent area.
3. Tubed Grafts (Indirect pedicle grafts) : It is indicated in those cases where the donor and the recipient area cannot be brought close to each other. It is done in stages. For example, tubed graft constructed from the abdomen is first attached to forearm and then it is finally put on the face.

10
Circumcision

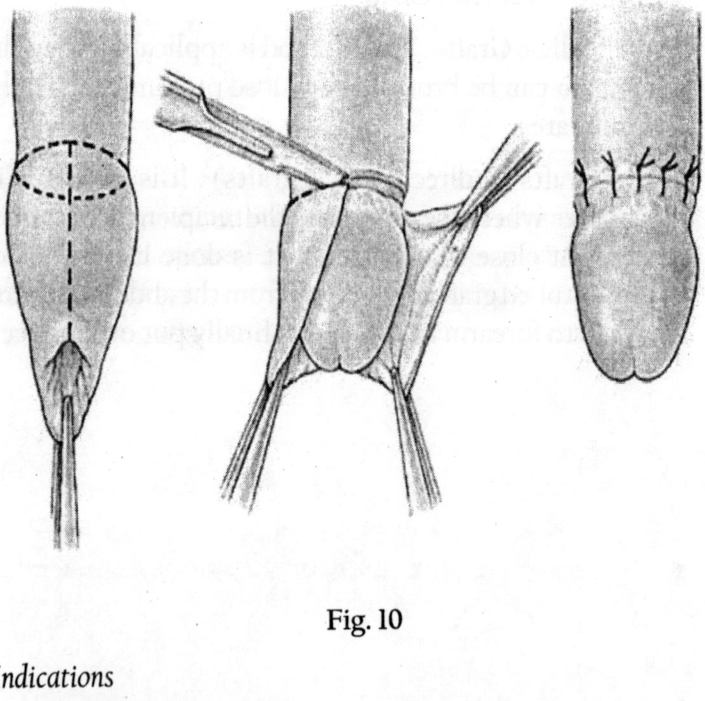

Fig. 10

Indications

1. For religious custom.
2. Phimosis.
3. Recurrent attacks of paraphimosis.
4. Recurrent attacks of balano-posthitis.

Anaesthesia:

General or Local.

Circumcision in Adult:

1. Separate the adhesions. if any, in between the prepuce and glans with the help of a probe or artery forceps.
2. Hold the margin of the prepuce in Allis/artery forceps.
3. Slit the prepuce in the mid-dorsal line beyond the middle of the glans.
4. Remove smegma.
5. Cut away the redundant parts of both prepucial layers in a line parallel to the corona (more of the inner layer being removed).
6. Catch the frenular artery; in the midline ventrally and secure it in 3 in 1 stitch (ligate it).
7. Ligate any other bleeding vessels.
8. Suture two layers of the prepucial skin by interrupted sutures (usually by Catgut).
9. Apply dressing (gauze) with ointment or tincture benzoin.

Circumcision in Child:

As the prepuce is long. an artery forceps is placed (clamped) across it just beyond the tip of the glans in an oblique line parallel to the corona. The prepuce beyond is cut off close to the clamp. The clamp is then removed. Other stages are the same as mentioned above.

The frenular artery must be adequately secured (tied), as sometimes, it may cause troublesome bleeding, contraindication of circumcision is hypospadius.

11
Vasectomy

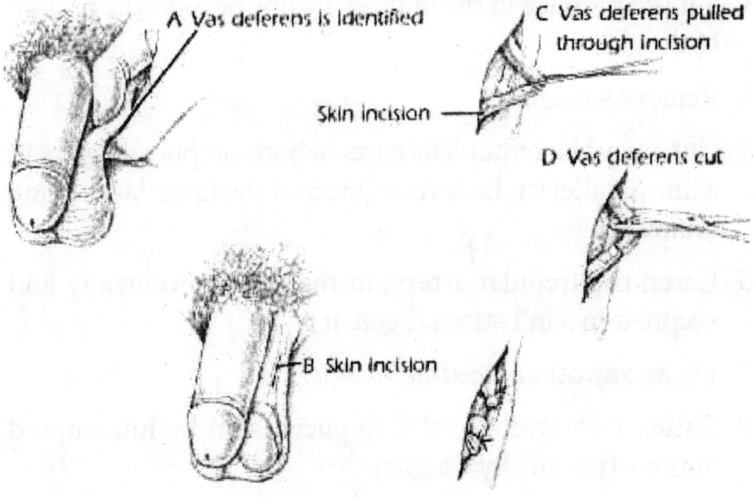

Fig. 11

Indications:

1. To effect sterilisation.
2. In association with prostatectomy to avoid epididymitis.

Anaesthesia:

Local.

Procedure:

1. Palpate the vas at the postero-lateral aspect of scrotum or near the root of penis (feels like cord).

2. Fix it with thumb and fingers.
3. Infiltrate L.A.
4. Transverse incision-about 1/2 to 1 inch.
5. Cut the layers-blunt dissection.
6. Catch the vas with Allis forceps.
7. Separate it from its coverings.
8. Divide between clamped forceps (a small portion may be removed).
9. Ligate the ends with silk.
10. Close the wound.

Complications:

Haematoma

Infection.

F.B. granuloma (or sperm granuloma).

12
Hyderocele

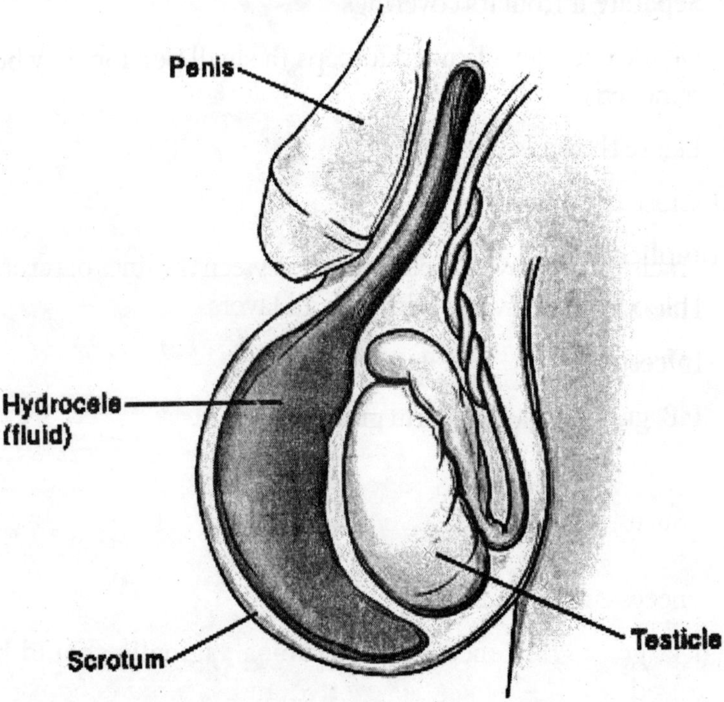

Fig. 12

Layers of Scrotum:

Skin, dartos, external spermatic fascia, cremasteric muscle and fascia, internal spermatic fascia, parietal layer of tunica vaginais.

Indications:

Hydrocele: pyocele, haematocele.

Anaesthesia:

General or Local.

Local anaesthesia usually preferred.

Procedure:

1. Cord block is done by injecting about 2 to 3 cc of 1% Xylocaine in the cord.
2. Assistant makes the hydrocele tense.
3. Infiltrate L. A. through all the layers.
4. Incision: Transverse/ oblique in between the lines of scrotal blood vessels (veins) through all layers.
5. Dissect and deliver the hydrocele.
6. Open the sac, drain the fluid, avoid injury to testis.
7. Evert the sac.
8. Suture the cut edge of tunica for haemostasis with catgut so that the sac remains everted. A few sutures may be necessary to retain it in position:

(If large or thickened, part of tunica vaginalis should be excised and the remainder everted and sutured behind the testis).

9. The margins of the sac should not be too tight around the cord (to avoid strangulation).
10. Secure haemostasis.
11. Close the wound.

Sometimes corrugated drain may be put in to avoid haematoma formation.

Complications:

Haematoma

Wound infection

Wound disruption.

13

Inguinal Hernia

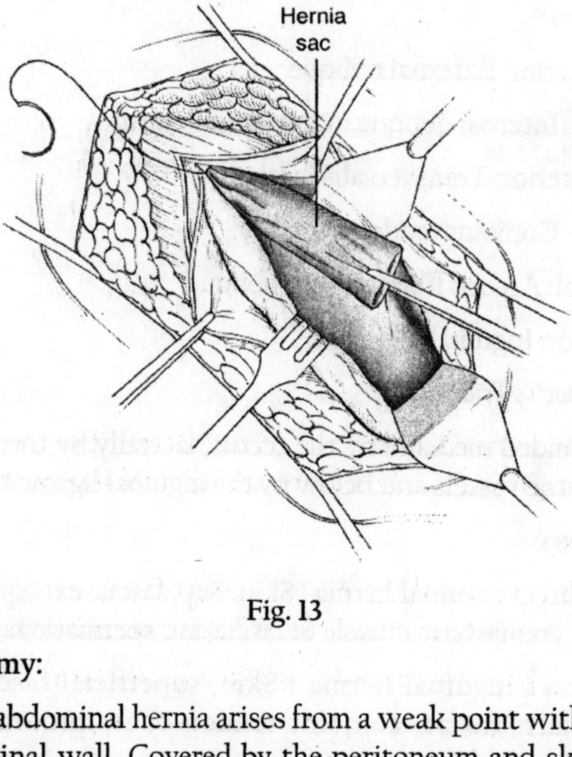

Fig. 13

Anatomy:

An abdominal hernia arises from a weak point within the abdominal wall. Covered by the peritoneum and skin, the abdominal organs (most of the times gut and fatty tissue) bulge through a gap between the muscles and the connective tissue. If the abdominal hernia arises above the groin ligament, it is called groin rupture (hernia inguinalis). In case of a hernia below the inguinal ligament, it is called femoral rupture (hernia femoralis). The inguinal as well as the femoral hernia are inherent weak spots within the tissue, which by time extend until a hole gapes open within the tissue. Length of inguinal canal is 1 and half inch, ext. inguinal ring lies just above the pubic tubercle.

Deep inguinal ring: lies half inch above the mid inguinal point.

Boundary:

Anterior: External oblique

Internal oblique in the lateral· third.

Posterior: Transversalis fascia

Conjoint tendon medially.

Roof: Arched fibres of into oblique.

Floor: Inguinal ligament.

Hesselbach's Triangle:

Bounded medially by the rectus, laterally by the inferior eptgastnc vessels and below by the inguinal ligament.

Coverings:

Indirect inguinal hernia ; Skin, Sup. fascia, ext. spermatic fascia, cremasteric muscle & fascia, int. spermatic fascia.

Direct inguinal hernia : Skin, superficial fascia, ext. spermatic fascia, conjoint tendon or its prolongation, transversalis fascia.

Under 3 years of age, both rings, lie superimposed.

Definitions:

I. Herniotomy : (Excision of the sac) Infant & children upto 14 years.

II. Herniorrhaphy: Young adult.

Excision of sac and repair of post. walf by absorbable or non-absorbable suture material e.g. catgut, thread, prolene,silk.

III. Hernioplasty: Excision of sac and repair of posterior wall by living material e.g. ext. oblique aponeurosis, fascia lata, skin ribbon.

Operative Procedure:

The essentials of hernia repair are:

a. Excision of sac (herniotomy):

b. Repair of posterior wall e.g. Conjoint tendon- Inguinal Ligament apposition (C.I.A.).

Steps of operation:

1. Inguinal incision about 1" above and parallel to medial 2/3 of inguinal ligament.
2. Cut skin & superficial fascia.
3. Cut ext. oblique-open superficial inguinal ring.
4. Raise the leaves of ext. oblique to define conjoint tendon medially and inguinal ligament laterally.
5. Visualise the Sac lying anterior to the cord, covered by cremasteric muscle & fascia.
6. Incise the coverings longitudinally define the sac as a pearly white structure, dissect and separate the sac from cord upto the neck.
7. Define the neck by finding extraperitoneal fat and inferior epigastric artery.
8. Transfix and ligate the neck, excise excess portion (Herniotomy).
9. Lift the cord on the sling.
10. Repair (stitch the conjoint tendon to the inguinal ligament) with a Ship of ext. oblique aponeurosis (hernioplasty) or prolene or by simple interrupted suture (Bassini's repair).

The most medial suture should include the periosterum of the pubic tubercle. While applying the suture, the bite on the inguinal ligament should be superficial so that the femoral vein is not punctured.

Some Surgeons prefer to do lytle's repair (narrowing the internal ring with lateral displacement of cord) specially of transversalis fascia (plication).

Shouldice repair consist of double breasting of transversalis fascia.

Tanner slide operation consists of relaxing incision of the, rectus sheath, after the repair of posterior wall.

Direct Inguinal Hernia:

Steps of operation are the same as those of an indirect hernia. In direct hernia, the sac is dissected free from the surrounding. structures & inverted into the abdomen by plication. Care is taken not to injure urinary bladder.

Sometimes if it is wide necked one, it is better to cut away the redundant portion & repair the sac (peritoneum) by continuous suture.

This is followed by repair as described for indirect hernia.

Sliding Hernia (Hernie-en-Glissade):

Steps of operation is the same as that of indirect hernia but no attempt should be made to dissect the caecum, sigmoid or urinary bladder (forming the posterior wall of the sac) free from the peritoneum otherwise the blood supply will be imperiled and it may lead to peritonitis or fistula. Only the free portion of the sac below the attached viscous is removed and the sac (peritoneum) is repaired by continuous suture and the whole mass is returned to the abdomen.

Orchidectomy in Hernia Operation

Orchidectomy should be considered while repairing hernia in elderly patients, recurrent hernia, sliding hernia or a very big hernia with very weak abdominal musculature.

Complications of Hernia Operation on the table:

a. Division of vas

b. Injury to deep epigastric vessels or

c. Injury to External iliac vessels.

Post-operative:

Haematoma, wound infection & recurrence.

14

Strangulated Inguinal Hernia

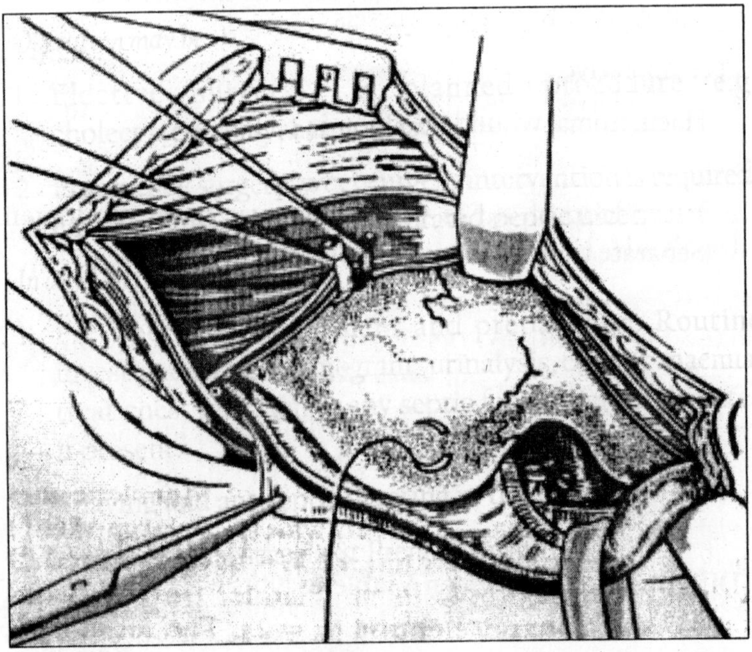

Fig. 14

Emergency Operation: Ryle's tube aspiration, intravenous fluids & antibiotics are absolutely essential.

Procedure: Preferably general anaesthesia.

1. Inguinal incision extending over the most prominent part of swelling.

2. Cut skin, superficial fascia, define External oblique aponeurosis & the sac with coverings.
3. Incise the coverings of the anterior surface of sac.
4. Incise the sac & drain out the toxic infected fluid.
5. Cut the constriction band & external oblique. Constriction band, in order of frequency, is located (a) At the superficial inguinal ring (b) In the inguinal canal (*c*) At the deep inguinal ring. At or near the deep ring the band should be incised parallel to the deep epigastric vessels i.e. upwards & medially.
6. Examine carefully the contents of the sac. Excise devitalised omentum after ligation (transfixation).
7. If the loop of gut is viable, return it to the abdomen. Separate the sac from its coverings.
8. Ligate (transfix) the neck of the sac: Herniotomy.
9. If the condition of the patient permits, repair the posterior wall as usual: Herniorrhaphy or Hernioplasty.

In doubtful cases warm moist abdominal pack should be applied many a times for atleast ten minutes to see if signs of viability set in.

Differentiation between Viable & Non-Viable loop:

Viable	*Non-Viable*
a. Dark colour becomes lighter.	a. Greenish or blackish in colour.
b. Presence of pulsation in the mesentery.	b. Pulsation absent.
c. Presence of peristalsis in the loop.	c. Peristalsis absent.
d. Peritoneum shiny.	d. Peritoneum dull and lustreless.

If the loop of the bowel is non-viable (gangrenous), Resection & anastomosis has to be performed.

Intestinal Resection and Anastomosis

Common indications:

1. Gangrene of a loop of bowel.
2. Trauma (irreparable injury).
3. Stricture e.g. Tuberculous.
4. Tumour: usually malignant tumour.

Anastomosis between the two ends is done in two layers.

a. 1st layer consisting of whole thickness.

b. 2nd layer consisting of seromuscular suture.

After anastomosis, mesentery of the two anastomosed ends are approximated.

Different methods

a. End to end

b. Side to side e.g. in Iliotransverse colostomy

c. End to side.

15
Femoral Hernia

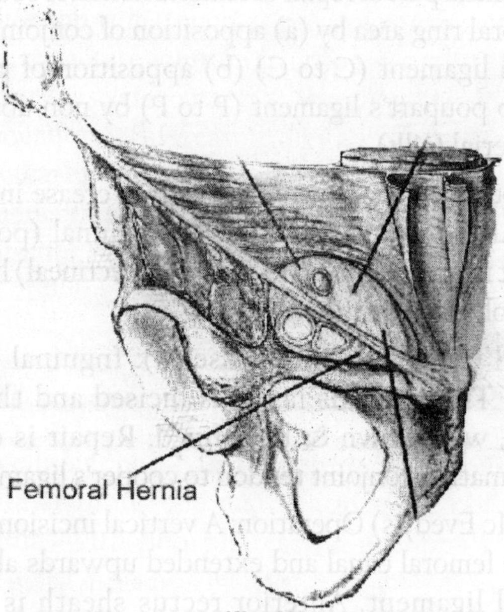

Fig. 15

Surgical Anatomy:

The femoral canal occupies the most medial compartment of the femoral sheath. It is about 1.25 cm long and 1.25 cm wide at the femoral ring. It contains fat, lymphatic vessels, and the gland of cloquet. It is most commonly found in females.

Boundaries of Femoral Ring:

Anterior: Inguinal (poupart's) ligament.

Posterior: Cooper's (pectineal) ligament.

Medial: Girnbernat's ligament.

Lateral: Septum separating it from the femoral vein.

Procedure:

Femoral hernias are very susceptible to strangulation because of the unyielding margins of the femoral ring e.g. knife like edge of Gimbernat's ligament.

The essential part of repair of femoral hernia is obliteration of the femoral ring area by (a) apposition of conjoint tendon to cooper's ligament (C to C) (b) apposition of pectineal ligament to poupart's ligament (P to P) by non-absorbable suture material (silk).

a. Low Operation (Lookwood's): A groin crease incision is made. After dcaling with the sac, inguinal (poupart's) ligament is approximated to cooper's (pectineal) ligament, so as to obliterate the femoral ring.

b. Inguinal Operation (Lotheissen's): Inguinal canal is opened. Transversalis fascia is incised and the sac is defined, withdrawn & transfixed. Repair is done by approximating conjoint tendon to cooper's ligament.

c. High (Mc Evedy's) Operation: A vertical incision is made over the femoral canal and extended upwards above the inguinal ligament. Anterior rectus sheath is incised vertically in its lowest part (medial to its lateral border). Rectus is retracted medially. Extraperitoneal space is cleared, sac is identified & withdrawn from the femoral canal & dealt. Repair is completed by apposing conjoint tendon to cooper's ligament.

For strangulated femoral hernia, Me Evedy's operation is preferable.

During repair of femoral hernia, care must be taken to protect external iliac/femoral vein on lateral side & urinary bladder on the medial side.

16
Umbilical Hernia

I. *Umbilical Hernia of Infants and Children:*

The vast majority close spontaneously during the first year of life. Strapping after putting a big coin or application of a rubber umbilical pad may encourage this process.

Where the hernia fails to disappear after the age of 2 years. operation is advised. Excision of the sac should be done through a semicircular subumbilical incision preserving the umbilicus. and the edges of the defect closed.

II. *Para Umbilical Hernia of Adults:*

Mayo's operation: Through a transverse elliptical incision umbilicus & hernial sac are excised. Rectus sheath is incised transversely on each side. Repair is done by overlapping (double- bracing) the edges of the rectus sheath above and below the hernia.

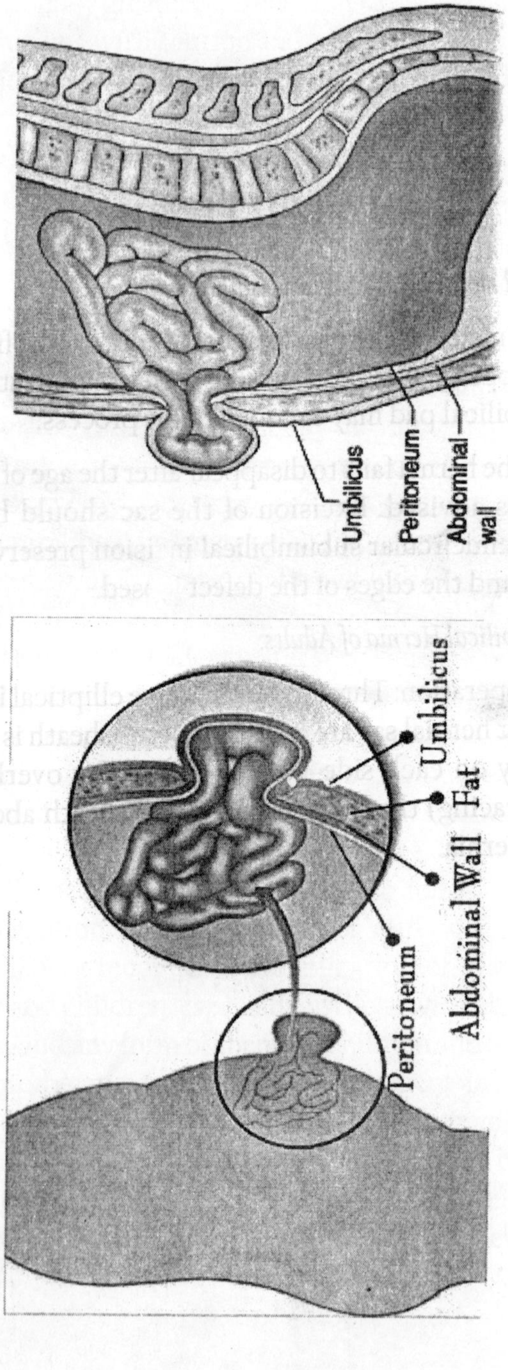
Umbilicus
Peritoneum
Abdominal wall
Umbilicus
Fat
Abdominal Wall
Peritoneum

Fig. 16

17
Appendicectomy

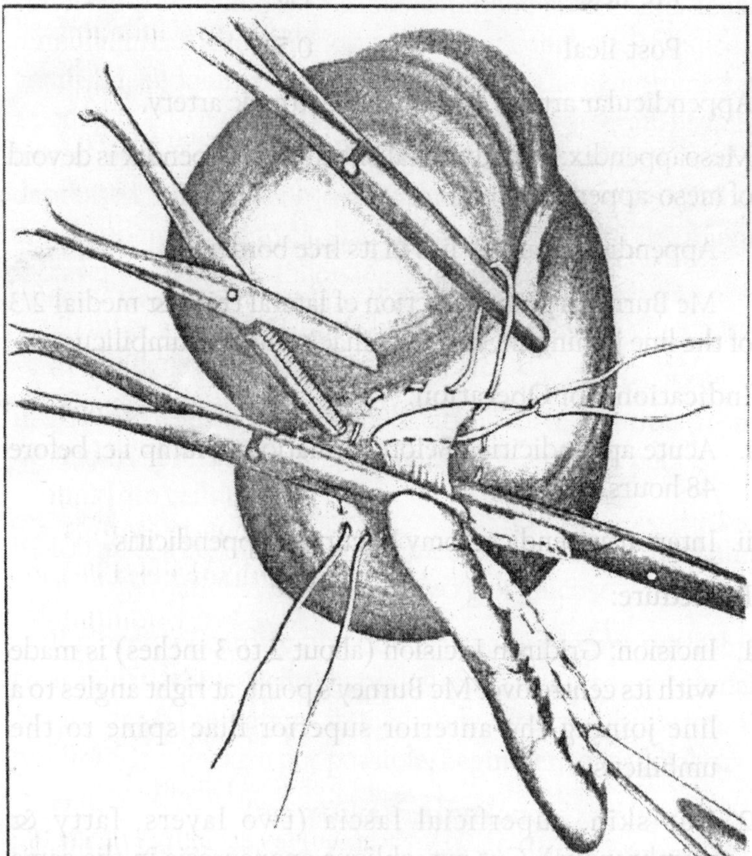

Fig. 17

Surgical Position:	**Anatomy: 6 to 10 cms in length**
Retrocaecal	74%
Pelvic	21%
Paracaccal	2%
Subcaecal	1.5%
Pre-ileal	1%
Post-ileal	0.5%

Appendicular artery: A branch of ileo colic artery.

Mesoappendix: Usually distal one third of appendix is devoid of meso-appendix.

Appendicular artery lies in its free border.

Me Burney's point: Junction of lateral third & medial 2/3 of the line joining the ant. sup. iliac spine and umbilicus.

Indications for Operation:

i. Acute appendicitis : Before formation of lump i.e. before 48 hours.

ii. Interval appendicectomy Recurrent appendicitis.

Procedure:

1. Incision: Gridiron Incision (about 2 to 3 inches) is made with its centre over Mc Burney's point, at right angles to a line joining the anterior superior iliac spine to the umbilicus.
2. Cut skin, superficial fascia (two layers, fatty & membranous). Cut ext. oblique aponeurosis in the same line.
3. Split fibres of int. oblique and tranversus. Apply retractors in the corners.

4. Lift the peritoneum with Allis forceps, open the peritoneum.
5. Search for the caecum and appendix (follow taenia coli to appendix).
6. Deliver caecum and appendix in the wound (catch the appendix with Allis' or Babcock's forceps).
7. Define mesoappendix, ligate & cut close to the appendicular attachment (Secure appendicular vessels).
8. Purse string suture (seromuscular) around the base in the caecum (with intestinal catgut).
9. Crush and ligate the base of appendix with thread (artery forceps holding the thread just adjacent to the knot). Remove the appendix.
10. Touch the stump with a swab (soaked in antiseptic solution).
11. Invaginate and tie the purse string suture. Inspect terminal ileum for any other pathology, look for haemostasis.
12. Closure: Close Peritoneum. Oppose split fibres of internal oblique & transversus. Suture ext. oblique -aponeurosis. Suture Skin.

Other Incisions:

1. Right paramedian.
2. Rutherford Morrison:(muscle cutting).
3. Lanz incision: Transverse in the inter spinous groove.

Some Important Considerations

1. In case of difficulty in tracing the appendix: *Try* to deliver the caecum & follow taenia coli. Enlarge incision by cutting the int. and transversus muscle.

2. If the base of the appendix is gangrenous: No purse string suture should be applied.

   Remove the appendix flush with the caecal wall.

   Close the defect in two layers.

3. Incidentally if it is a case of tuberculosis or Crohn's disease. Appendicectomy should be avotded for the fear of fistula formation.

4. In case of difficulty in finding the tip.

   Retrograde appendicectomy: deal the base first, invaginate and then remove the mesoappendix bit by bit till you reach the tip..

5. A drainage tube may be put in, in a case of ruptured appendix.

Post-Operative Complications:

1. Ileus.
2. Wound infection.
3. Residual abscess.
4. Faecal fistula.
5. Int. obstruction.
6. Pyelephlebitis.
7. Pulmonary complications.
8. Incisional hernia.

18

Abdominal Incisions

Paramedian:

1.	Right	Upper
	Left	Middle
		Lower
2.	Midline	Upper
		Lower

3. Subcostal Right (Kocher's) Left.
4. Grid-iron incision
5. Lanz incison
6. Battle incision (Para recta)).
7. Rutherford Morrison (Muscle cutting iliac incision).

Paramedian Incision

Upper: above umbilicus

Middle.

Lower: below umbilicus.

It is the most widely used incision.

Procedure:

1. Incision: Parallel to midline about 1" lateral to it.

2. Cut skin, superficial fascia.
3. Incise anterior rectus sheath in the line of skin incision.
4. Apply forceps on the medial cut edge of the rectus sheath.
5. Separate rectus muscle from the medial leaf and retract it laterally.

Three tendinous intersections : one at the level of umbilicus, one near Xiphisternum and one is between them. Tendinous intersections are not attached to the posterior sheath.

Nerve supply to rectus comes from lateral side.

6. Lift the posterior sheath, alongwith peritoneum and incise in the line of skin incision.

Closure: In three layers.

lst layer: Peritoneum and post. sheath.

2nd layer: Ant. rectus sheath.

3rd layer: Skin.

19
Peptic Ulcer

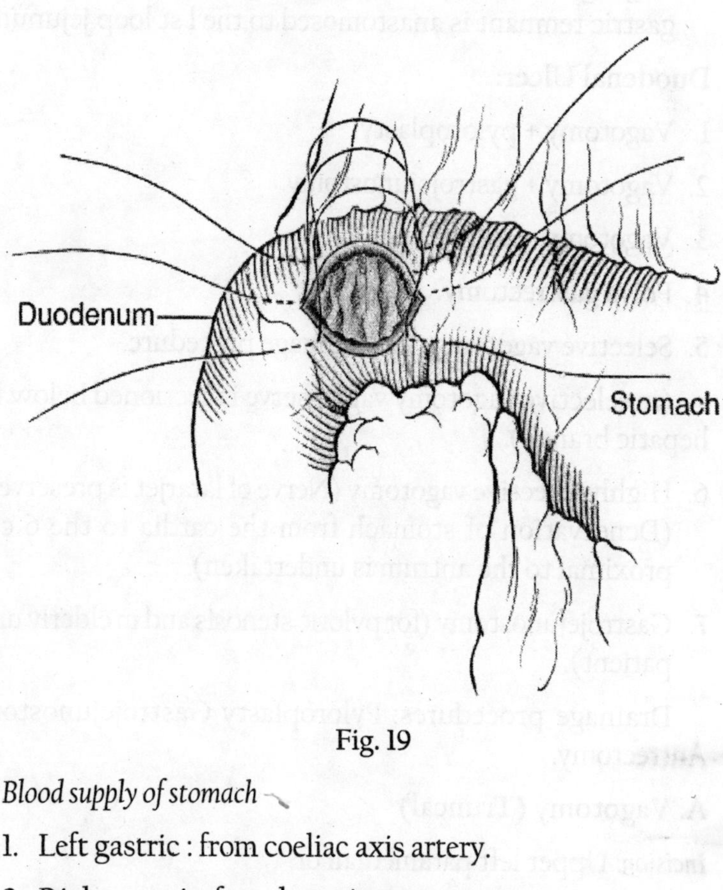

Fig. 19

Blood supply of stomach

1. Left gastric : from coeliac axis artery.
2. Right gastric: from hepatic artery.
3. Right gastroepiploic artery: from gastroduodenal artery.

4. Left gastroepiploic artery: from splenic artery.
5. Short gastric arteries from splenic artery.

Operations:

Gastric Ulcer: Partial gastrectomy

1. Billroth I-where gastroduodenal continuity is maintained.
2. Polya gastrectomy: Duodenal stump is closed, and the gastric remnant is anastomosed to the 1 st loop jejunum.

Duodenal Ulcer:

1. Vagotomy + pyloroplasty.
2. Vagotomy + gastrojcjunostomy.
3. Vagotomy + antrectomy
4. Polya gastrectomy.
5. Selective vagotomy plus drainage procedure.

(in selective vagotomy vagus nerve is sectioned below the hepatic branch).

6. Highly selective vagotomy (Nerve of latarjet is preserved). (Dcnervation of stomach from the cardia to the 6 cms proximal to the antrum is undertaken).
7. Gastrojejunostomy (for pyloric stenosis and in elderly unfit patient).

Drainage procedures: Pyloroplasty Gastrojejunostomy Antrectomy.

A. Vagotomy (Truncal)

Incision: Upper left paramedian or

Upper midline.

Procedure:

1. Confirm the diagnosis and pack off the transverse colon and small intestines downwards.

2. Retract the left lobe of liver and divide the left triangular ligament. (Avoidinjury to subdiaphragmatic veins).
3. With the help of deep retractors the gastro-oesophageal junction is brought into view:
4. Assistant pulls the stomach downwards alongwith the Ryle's tube, lying in the stomach.
5. Transverse incision in the peritoneum overlying the lower part of oesophagus.
6. Feel (usually visible) the anterior vagus as a taut cord and with blunt dissection define it with a long curved haemostat or Moynihan's forceps.
7. Cut the anterior vagus (Clamps may be applied).
8. Pass the right index finger, around the oesophagus to encircle it, feeling the Ryle's tube in the lumen, as a guide and let it emerge on the right side of hiatus.
9. Pass a rubber catheter around the oesophagus with the help of index finger (Loop of the catheter will be pulled out. This will act as a rectractor of the hiatus.
10. Feel the posterior vagus in the peri oesophageal tissue as a taut cord (thicker than anterior vagus) and hook it out.
11. Divide it in between the clamps. Ligate the cut ends.
12. Check for any remaining fibres and divide them.
13. Pack the area, complete the drainage procedure, remove the pack and look for haemostasis.

Complications:

Specific:

1. Transitory dysphagia
2. Gastric retention
3. Diarrhoea.

B. Gastrojejunostomy

1. Posterior (Retrocolic): to transverse colon.
2. Anterior (Antecolic): for carcinoma stomach as palliative procedure.

Indications:

1. In combination with vagotomy.
2. Pyloric obstruction : Pyloric stenosis, Carcinoma of stomach (as a palliative measure).

Incisions: Upper paramedian

Upper midline.

Procedure

1. Open the abdomen. Confirm diagnosis.
2. Lift transverse colon. Look for middle colic artery.
3. Incise avascular area in the transverse mesocolon lateral to the left branch of middle colic artery.
4. Pull out the stomach through the incised mesocolon.
5. Catch hold about 3-4" of stomach (in between the lesser and greater curvature) in intestinal clamp (gastric clamp).
6. Bring out the 1st loop of jejunum and catch hold the 3-4" of jejunum in intestinal clamp.
7. 1st layer of suture: seromuscular.
8. Open the stomach and jejunum parallel to the seromuscular suture.
9. Second layer: whole thickness of post. leaves of stomach and jejunum.
10. Third layer : whole thickness of ant. leaves of stomach and jejunum.

Partial Gastrectomy:

1. Incision is made extending from upper mid-abdomen to the belly button.
2. If this is done for ulcer disease, the nerves that control acid production may also be cut.
3. Separate mesocolon from the posterior wall of the stomach. (Take care not to injure middle colic vessels).
4. Define and divide right gastro-epiploic pedicles between ligatures; near the pylorus.
5. Define right gastric pedicle, by drawing the duodenum forward and downward, in the hepato gastric omentum, close to the upper border of duodenum. Divide it between; the ligatures (or clamps). Common bile duct should not be injured.
6. Hold the upper and lower border of duodenum with Allis' forceps. Clamp the pylorus with crushing clamp (or Payr's clamp).
7. Transect the duodenum close to the crushing clamp and tum the stomach alongwtth the clamp to the left.

Closure of duodenum:

a. Stitch the duodenal edges (the all-coats layer) with continuous stitch.

b. Invaginate the closed duodenal stump by means of seromuscular layer.

(As a final safeguard, the duodenal stump may be snugly buried by stitches between the anterior duodenal wall and the capsule of the pancreas).

1. Identify the left gastric pedicle. Ligate the descending branch of left gastric artery (Double ligatures preferred).
2. Clean the lesser curve for 2-3 cms. below this point.

3. Divide lower two or three short gastric vessels between ligatures and select the site of gastric transection. (The antecolic or retrocolic gastrojejunal anastomosis with or without valve is performed).
4. Antecolic gastrojejunal anastomosis: During the 1st loop of jejunum (about 3-4 inches from the duodenojejunal flexure) antertor to transverse colon and hold it in intestinal clamp (or preferably in the first of Lane's twin clamp).
5. Put posterior seromuscular suture of catgut.
6. Apply Payr's clamps across two thirds of the stomach. Apply Intestinal damp (or 2nd of Lanes's twin damp) across the stomach proximal to the seromuscular suture.
7. Transect the stomach by cutting close to the Payr's clamp. Valve may be constructed by means of continuous catgut suture commencing on the lesser curve.
8. Incise the jejunum opposite the open part of stomach about 1/4 inch, from the seromuscular suture.
9. Complete the posterior and anterior, all coats layer anastomosis, commencing at the lower end.
10. Complete the anterior seromuscular layer, incorporating the valve and the anastomosis with continuous suture.
11. Drainage tube may be put in dose to the duodenal stump.
12. Close the abdomen in layers.

D. Closure of Perforated Peptic Ulcer

Urgent operation after resuscitation is essential. General anaesthesia, supine postilion.

Incision:

Upper right paramedian.

Escape of gas and fluid after opening the peritoneum shows the correctness of the diagnosis.

Procedure: After opening the abdomen.

1. Suck the fluid or exudate from the peritoneal cavity (Supra colic compartment).
2. Search the site of perforation (in the duodenum or the stomach).
3. Insert Lembert sutures (usually 3-4) in the transverse axis of the organ and hole the ends of the catgut by haemostats (artery forceps).
4. Tie the knots firmly but not tightly.
5. Put omental patch to buttress the sutured perforation, and fix the patch with catgut.
6. Do peritoneal toilet.
7. Drainage tube may be put in. S. Closure in layers.

20

Right Hemicolectomy

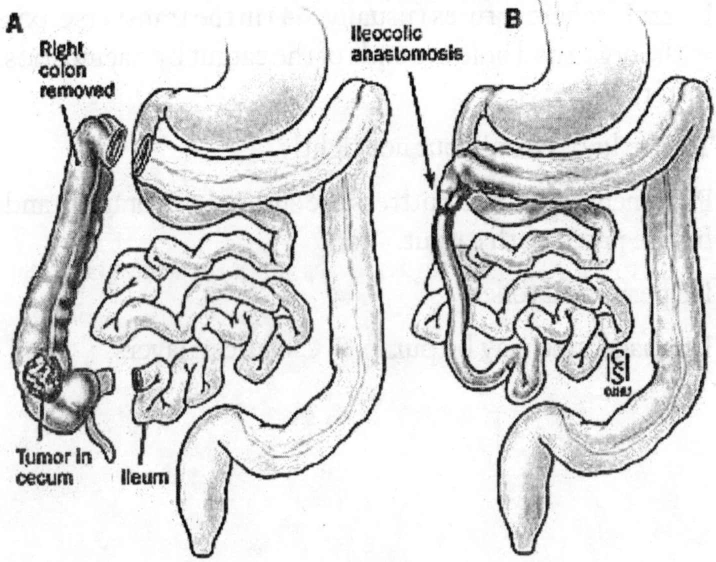

Fig. 20

Indications:

1. Carcinoma of the caecum or ascending colon.
2. Ileocaecal tuberculosis.
3. Carcinoid of terminal ileum.
4. Carcinoid of the Appendix involving the base.
5. An intussusception when the affected gut is damaged beyond recovery.

Structures removed:

Terminal 6 inches of the ileum, the caecum, the ascending colon and the proximal one third of the transverse colon.

Continuity is re-established by an ileo transverse anastomosis- Terminal 6 inches of ileum is removed as it is supplied by ileo-colic artery.

Injury to the duodenum & the Right ureter is avoided. Ileocolic & right colic vessels are ligated and divided.

Procedure:

Prepare bowel by giving oral Neomycin, Tinidazole & Enemata.

1. Right paramedian incision.
2. Confirm the diagnosis and operability of the lesion (In case the tumour is fixed with secondaries to liver or peritoneum, Ileo transverse colostomy should be done as a palliative procedure).
3. Mobilize right colon by incising the peritoneum along the lateral paracolic gutter down to the caecum and upto the hepatic flexure (it may involve division of the vessels in the right margin of the gastrocolic omentum between artery forceps).
4. Avoid injury to duodenum & right ureter.
5. Ligate & divide ileocolic and right colic vessels (The right branch of the middle colic artery is ligated and divided if an extensive resection is required for malignant disease, but often this vessel may be preserved).
6. Separate the greater omentum from the transverse colon upto and a few centimetres beyond the point of division of the transverse colon.
7. Divide the transverse colon & the ileum between clamps. Clean the cut ends with swabs.

(Ileum is divided obliquely making the anternescntertc border shorter than the mesentric border to obtain extra width).

8. Check for the vascularity (Cut ends of intestines should bleed freely after releasing the intestinal clamps).
9. Perform anastomosis in two layers (a) First layer-all coat sutures using continuous I/O or 2/0 atraumatic catgut. (b) 2nd layer- Scromuscular interrupted sutures using atraumatic 2/0 thread or silk.
10. Close the mesenteric gap carefully, using interrupted 2/0 atraumatic thread/catgut sutures.
11. Closures of abdomen in layers.

Complications:

Besides general complications, specific complications include primary and reactionary haemorrhage, wound infection, wound disruption, ileus and anastomotic leakage with subsequent peritonitis.

21
Colostomy

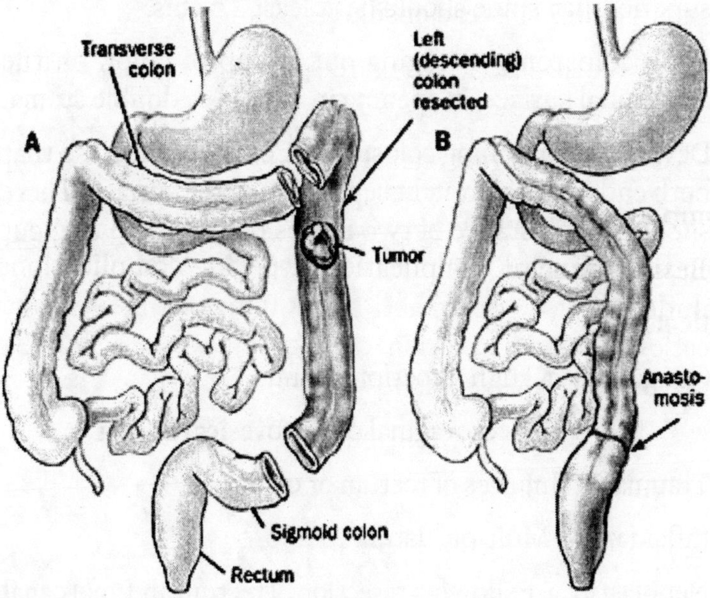

Fig. 21

Colostomy is an artificial opening made into the colon in order to divert faeces and flatus to the exterior.

I. A colostomy may be:

1. Temporary: e.g. in cases of acute obstruction.
2. Permanent: e.g. after abdominoperineal excision, Excision of carcinoma of rectum and anal canal.

II. Depending upon the site, a colostomy may be

a. Pelvic colostomy

b. Transverse colostomy.

III. Colostomy may be

1. Terminal colostomy: Bringing out the terminal end of colon on the abdomen, as in cases of carcinoma rectum. There is a single stoma. Distance of the stoma from the anterior superior iliac spine should be at least 2.5 cms.

2. Loop colostomy: Bringing out a loop of colon on the abdominal surface & opening it. There is a double stoma.

3. Devine defunctioning colostomy: Colon is divided so that both ends can be brought separately to the surface. There should be a distance of two inches between the two cut ends of the colon.

Indications:

1. Congenital a. High imperforate anus.

   b. Rectovaginal or rectovesical fistula.

2. Traumatic: Injuries of rectum or colon.

3. Inflamatory: Multiple fistula-in-ano,

4. Neoplastic: a. Following resection of rectum and anal canal (operable or inoperable).

   b. Preparatory procedure prior to resection of left colon or rectum.

Complications of colostomy include- Retraction, prolapse, stenosis, incisional hernia, sloughing, lateral space obstruction (due to failure to obliterate the lateral space between the colon & parietal wall) and Perforation (from an enema tube).

22
Cholecystectomy

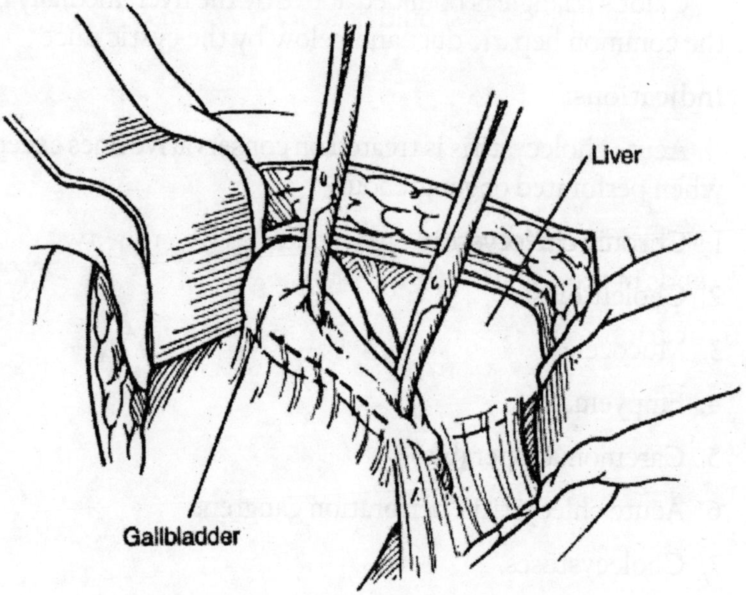

Fig. 22

Surgical anatomy G.B.-7.5 to 12.5 ems long (3"-5").

Cystic duct- 2.5 ems (1") CBD- 7.5 ems (3") CHD- 2.5 ems (1")

Parts: Fundus, body, neck, angulated distal part

Hartman's pouch and cystic duct.

Arterial supply : Cystic artery, a branch from right hepatic artery usually passing above and behind the cystic duct.

CBD:

Supra duodenal, retroduodenal, infraduodenal and intraduodenal portion.

Junction of cystic and common hepatic duct-T junction. There may be various types of congenital anomalies of gall bladder cystic duct and cystic artery.

Calot's triangle is bounded above by the liver, medially by the common hepatic duet and below by the cystic duct.

Indications:

Acute cholecystitis is treated on conservative lines except when perforated or gangrenous.

1. Chronic cholecystitis
2. Cholelithiasis
3. Mucocele
4. Empyema
5. Carcinoma (operable)
6. Acute chlecystitis: perforation gangrene
7. Cholecystoses.

Incision: Upper (R) paramedian

Transverse incision

Subcostal (Kocher's)incision.

Procedure:

1. Confirm the diagnosis
2. Isolate the area, one pack over the transverse colon and duodenum, another pack over the stomach.
3. Catch the fundus with a long haemostat or cholecystectomy clamp-acting as retractor.

4. Dissect and define the cystic duct and T junction, usually by blunt dissection with cholecystectomy clamp.
5. Catch the Hartman's pouch with another pair of haemostat.
6. Pass ligature around the cystic duct, tie and divide it in between the clamps and ligated end. Take care to leave considerable amount of cystic duct stump so that the ligature *may* not slip out.
7. Define cystic artery, divide it between ligature and clamp.
8. Beware of any accessory artery, any congenital anomaly and about bleeding.
9. Separate gall bladder from the liver bed by cutting the leaves of peritoneum on either side of gall bladder.
10. In the end leave the separated gall bladder to act as retractor.
11. Peritonealise the raw area of liver by stitching the cut edges of peritoneum.
12. Remove the gall bladder.
13. Put in a drianage tube through a separate stab wound in the right flank.
14. Close the abdomen.

Indications for exploration of Common Bile Duct:

1. Jaundice or history of jaundice.
2. Stone in C.B.D.
3. Dilated C.B.D. (more than 10 mms).
4. Gall bladder filled with small multiple stones.
5. Single faceted stone' in the gall bladder.
6. Wall of C.B.D. enormously thickened.
7. Negative shadow in operative cholangiography.

23

Choledocholithotomy (Supraduodenal)

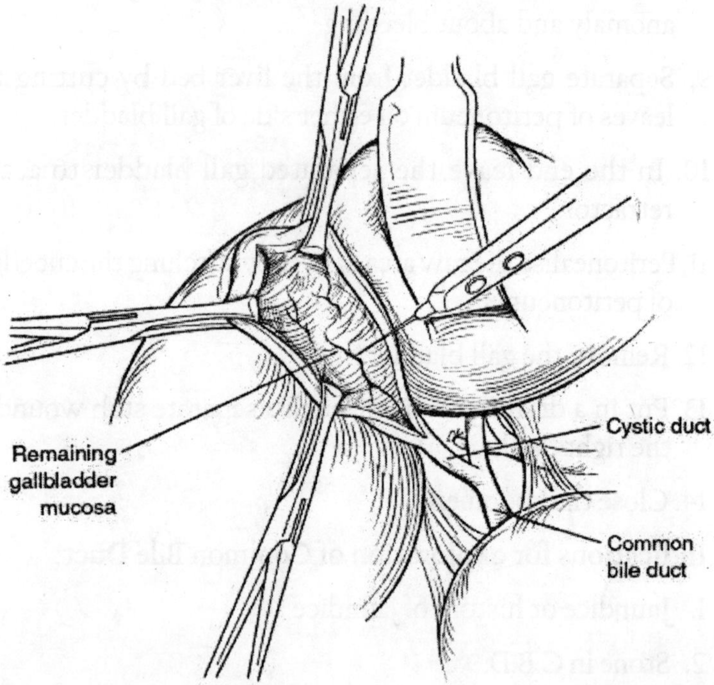

Preoperative preparation:

1. Plenty of intravenous Dextrose (10%) : to make good the liver insufficiency (3-4 days prior to surgery).

2. Vito K (parenteral) daily at least 3-4 days prior to surgery for maintaining normal prothrombin level in the blood.
3. Correction of anaemia.
4. Antibiotics to control the biliary infection.

Procedure:

1. Identify CBD at the right free margin of epiploic foramen (foramen of Winslow). In cases of doubt, aspirate bile by means of fine needle.
2. Apply two stay sutures on the CBD in vertical axis.
3. Incise CBD in between the sutures, milk out stone/stones through the choledochotomy incision or remove the stone by Desjardins forceps, malleable scoop or with the help of fogarty catheter.
4. Pass urethral bougie of suitable size upwards and also downwards till tip is felt inside the second part of duodenum.
5. Flush out any possible debris or gravels by saline water through a catheter.
6. Introduce T-tube of suitable size (after testing its patency & cutting the excess portions of transverse limb) into the duct. Suture the excess of the opening, in the duct by the side of the T-tube.

T-tube is usually removed in about 7-10 days time, provided intermittent & continuous clamping does not produce pain or leakage of bile around the tube, colour of stool should be of normal colour (not pale or white). T-tube cholangiogram must show free passage of dye into the duodenum without any negative shadow.

Post-operative complications include:

Haemorrhage, injury to CBD, or duodenum, ileus, peritonitis, pancreatitis, pyelephlcbitis, wound infection, biliary fistula etc.

24

Spleenectomy

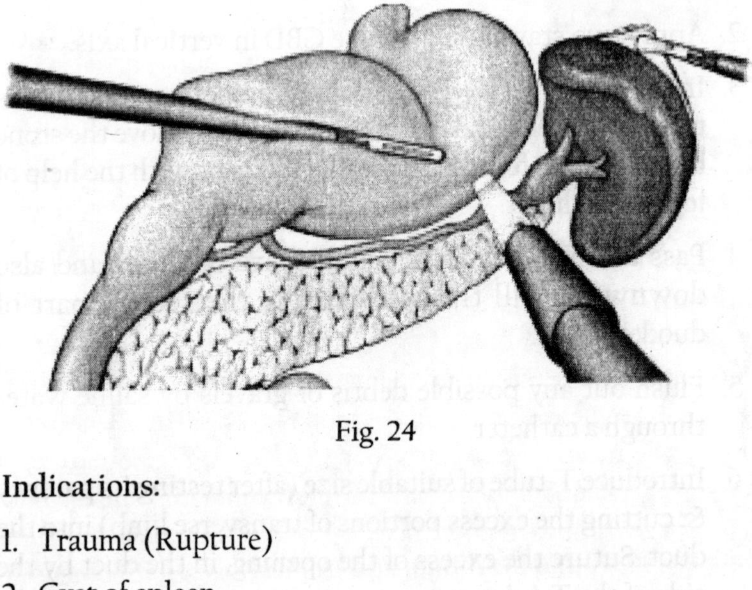

Fig. 24

Indications:

1. Trauma (Rupture)
2. Cyst of spleen
3. Acholuric jaundice
4. Hodgkin's disease (staging)
5. Preparation for Lieno renal anastomosis
6. Thrombocytopenic purpura
7. Tumour
8. Thallasserma

9. Torsion.

Anaesthesia:

General.

Position:

Supine.

Procedure:

Mobilize and rotate the spleen medially in the wound. Separate vascular adhesions, if any. Incise lateral peritoneum to expose lieno-renal ligament. Separate the tail of pancreas. Divide and transfix the lieno-renal pedicle.

Deal with the gastrosplenic ligament.

For non-traumatic cases:

First deal with gastrosplenic ligament. Then the vessels in the lieno-renal ligamens are dissected out, ligated and divided.

A drainage tube is put in.

Complications:

I. General: cardiac, pulmonary or thrombotic.

II. Injury to the tail of pancreas, fundus, haemorrhage.

III. Sepsis, wound dtsrupuon, peritonitis.

IV. Abdominal pain with fever, thrombosis of portal vein.

V. Postsplenectomy septicaemia-mainly due to meningococcal.

25

Lumbar Sympathectomy

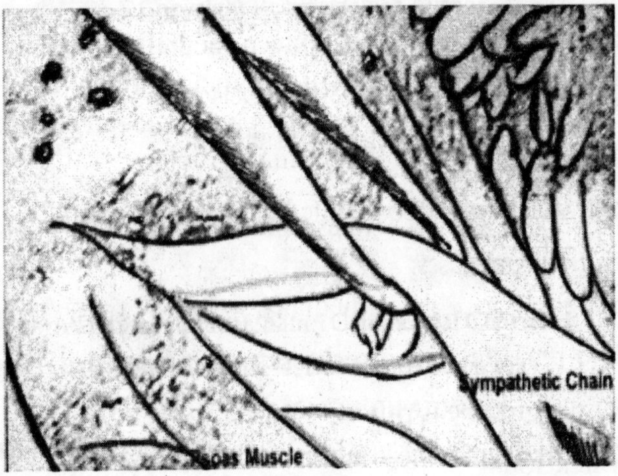

Fig. 25

The main aim of the lumbar sympathectomy should be to improve the blood flow to the skin vessels by protecting them against arteriospasm. However the indications are :

1. Hyperhidrosis.
2. Certain types of obscure pain such as causalgia.
3. Vasospastic conditions.
4. Buerger's disease and other peripheral arteritis.
5. To improve skin nutrition (healing of ischaemic ulcers).
6. In conjunction with direct arterial surgery, if the run off is poor.

7. To lower the level of amputation.

Anaesthesia:

General.

Position:

Semiprone.

Incision:

Transverse or oblique loin incision (from a point below the tip of 12th rib to the border of rectus).

Procedure:

Cut skin, sup. fascia, ext. & int. oblique and transversus.

1. Take care not to open the peritoneum.
2. Strip the peritoneum medially so as to expose the inner border of the psoas muscle (ureter and genital vessels being raised with it).
3. Search for the sympathetic chain lying in the groove between the vertebral bodies and the' psoas muscle, over- lapped by the vena cava on the right side and aorta on the left side.
4. Divide (or avulse) the sympathetic trunk and remove 2nd, 3rd & 4th ganglia.

(1st ganglion lies under the crus of the diaphragm, bilateral removal will lead to impotency).

5. Avoid injury (tearing off) of lumbar veins.

Care should be taken not to mistake lymph nodes, genitofemoral nerve and psoas minor muscle (if present) for the sympathetic chain.

6. Closure: Muscles in two layers.

   Followed by suture of the skin.

26

Haemorrhoidectomy

Treatment of Haemorrhoids

1. Injection 1 st degree & early 2nd degree haemorrhoids, 5% Phenol in almond oil (by Gabriel's syringe 3-5 ml).
2. Anal stretching (Lord's procedure).
3. Banding treatment (for 2nd degree) by Baron's Bands.
4. Cryo surgery.

Indications of Haemorrhoidectomy:

1. 3rd degree haemorrhoids.
2. Late 2nd degree haemorrhoids.
3. Fibrosed haemorrhoids.
4. Intero external haemorrhoids when the external haemorrhoid is well defined.

Haemorrhoidectomy:

Preparation:

a. Laxative 36 to 48 hours before operation.

b. Liquid or non residue diet.

c. Enema & bowel wash on the evening before operation or early in the morning.

d. Intestinal antiseptic may be given for 48 hours prior to surgery, e.g. Neomycin, Tinidazole.

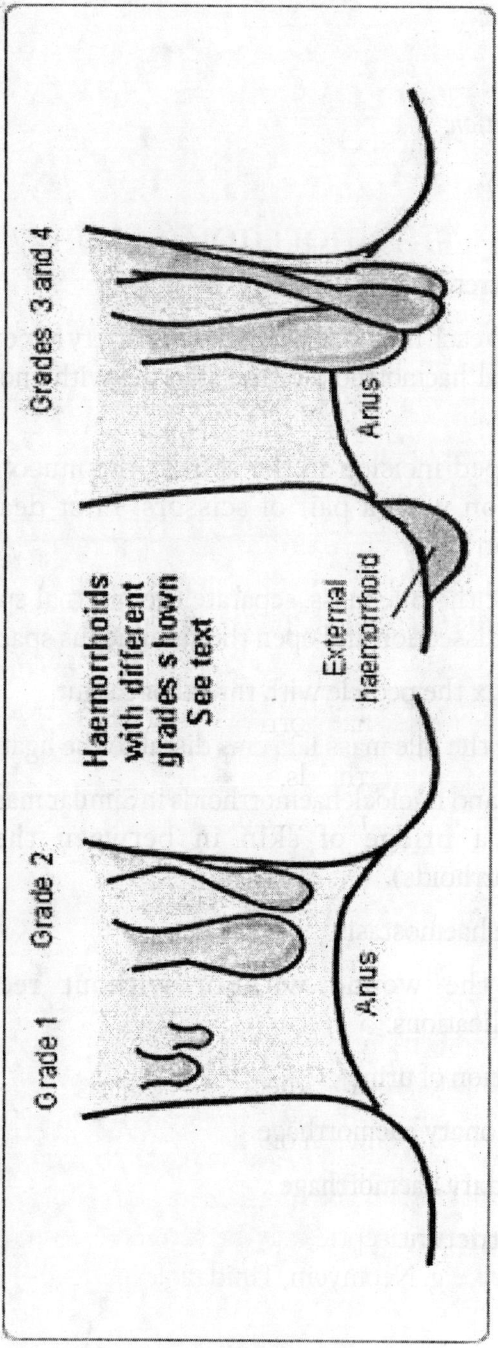
Grade 1
Grade 2
Grades 3 and 4
Haemorrhoids with different grades s hown See text
Anus
Anus
External haemorrhoid

Fig. 26

Anaesthesia:

General

Spinal Position:

Lithotomy.

Procedure:

1. Anal stretching is done.
2. Pick up each haemorrhoid mass with artery forceps, hold the external haemorrhoid or the skin tag with another artery forceps.
3. V shaped incision in the skin at the muco cutaneous junction with a pair of scissors. First deal 3° clock haemorrhoid.
4. Dissect the pile mass, separate the internal sphincter by blunt dissection and open the submucous space.
5. Transfix the pedicle with thread or catgut.
6. Excise the pile mass 1.25 cms distal to the ligature.
7. Deal 7 and 11° clock haemorrhoids in Similar manner (must leave a bridge of skin in between the excised haemorrhoids).
8. Secure haemostasis.
9. Pack the wound with or without rectal tube. Complications:

a. Retention of urine
b. Reactionary haemorrhage
c. Secondary haemorrhage
d. Anal stricture.

27

Suprapubic Cystostomy

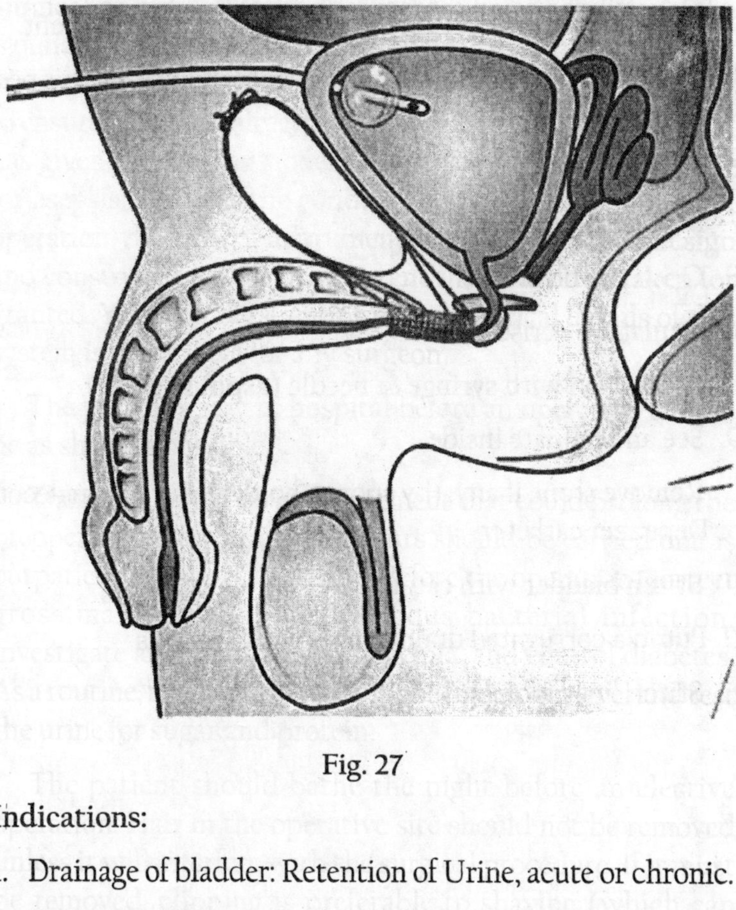

Fig. 27

Indications:

1. Drainage of bladder: Retention of Urine, acute or chronic.
2. For treating intra vesical pathology e.g. stone-suprapubic cystolithotomy, growth, diverticula.

3. For transvestcal (Freyer's) prostatectomy.

Steps:

1. Incision: Lower midline or tranverse just above pubis.
2. Out skin, subcutaneous tissue and
3. Linea alba (Ant. rectus sheath).
4. Separate Rectus muscles & Pyramidalis to expose transversalis fascia. Posterior rectus sheath is deficient.
5. Overlying peritoneum with the extraperitoneal fat stripped upwards.
6. Recognise bladder - by veins
7. Stay sutures.
8. Open the bladder.

Musculature - criscross

Aspiration with syringe & needle (aspirate urine).

9. See and palpate inside.

Remove stone if any, (by sponge holder). Put in a malecot or Depezzer catheter.

10. Stitch bladder with catgut.
11. Put in a corrugated drain in the cave of retzius.
12. Stitch linea alba & skin.

28
Prostatectomy

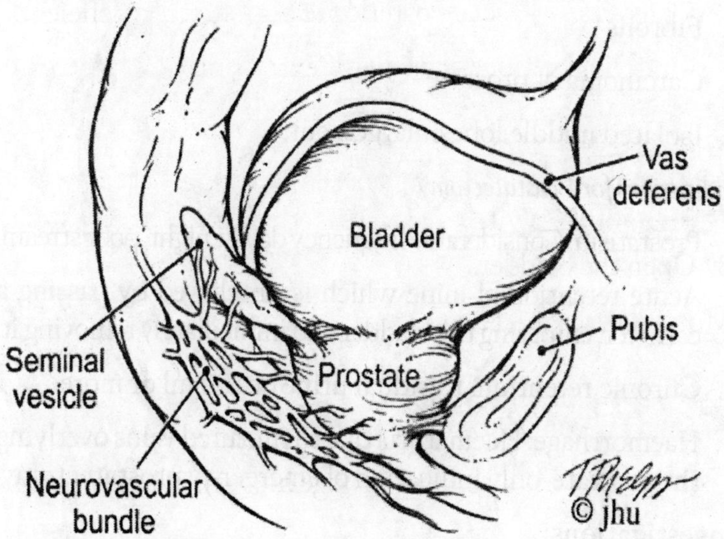

Fig. 28

1. Transvesical (Freyer's)

1st stage

2nd stage

Procedure:

When the renal function is poor or suprapubic cystostomy has been done for acute retention.

1st stage: suprapubic

2nd stage: removal of prostatic adenoma.

2. Retropubic (Millin's).
3. Perineal (Young's).
4. Transurethral prostate resection T.U.R.

Main indications are:

a. Fibrous
b. Carcinoma of prostate
c. Isolated middle lobe enlargement.

Indications for Prostatectomy

1. Prostatism: Considerable frequency day & night, poor stream.
2. Acute retention of mine which is unrelieved by passing a catheter, emptying the bladder and immediately removing it.
3. Chronic retention: Residual urine of 200 ml or more.
4. Haemorrhage: Haematuria due to ruptured veins overlying the prostate-only indication of emergency prostatectomy.

Investigations:

1. Routine investigations, urine culture & sensitivity.
2. Blood urea & creatinine.
3. I.V.P. & post micturition cystogram.
4. Serum acid phosphatase (Normal 1-3 king Armstrong units).
5. Ultrasonogram (Transrectal).
6. Cystoscopy: if Millin's prostatectomy is planned.
7. P.S.A. (Prostate specific antigen).

29

Exposure of the Kidney

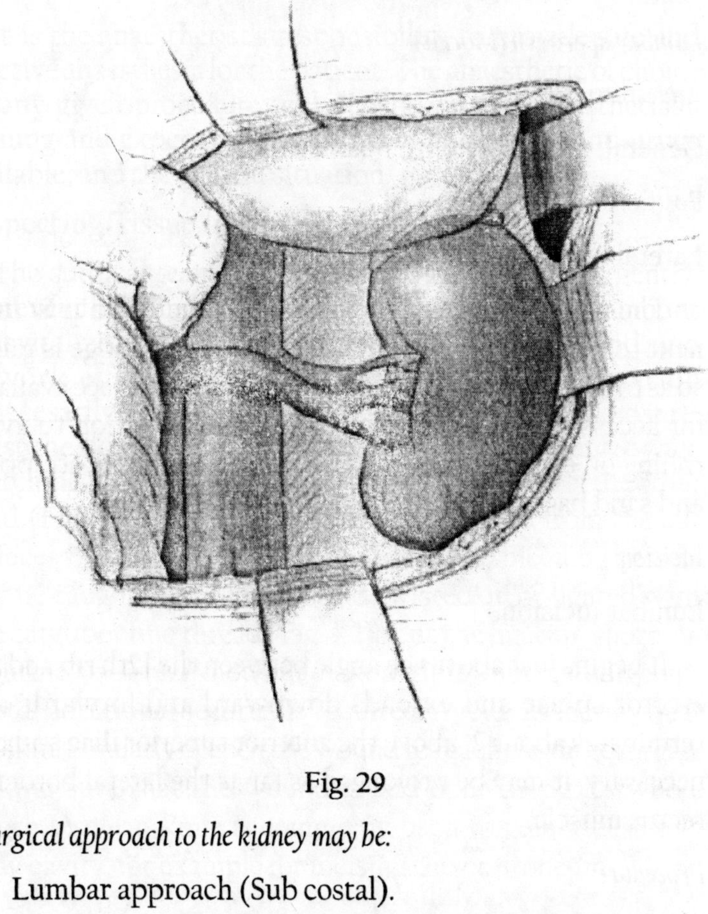

Fig. 29

Surgical approach to the kidney may be:

1. Lumbar approach (Sub costal).
2. Through the bed of the 12th rib (Transcostal).

3. Throraco abdominal approach (Through the bed of the 10th rib).
4. Transperitoneal approach.

Lumbar approach is most commonly employed. It is entirely extraperitoneal. The transperitoneal approach should be preferred in the case of renal tumours, as the pedicle can be dealt with, before the kidney is manipulated and the risk of spread of malignant cells is controlled.

Lumbar approach (Morris)

Anaesthesia:

General, preferably with relaxant.

Position:

Lateral kidney position.

The patient is placed on his sound side. The hip & knee next to the table are fully flexed. The kidney bridge is raised so as to flex the trunk laterally and increase the space available for access. The patient is secured in this position to avoid rolling on either side by a broad band of adhesive strapping and sand bags.

Incision:

Lumbar incision.

It begins just above the angle between the 12th rib and the erector spinae and extends downward and forwards and terminates about 2" above the anterior superior iliac spine. If necessary, it may be prolonged as far as the lateral border of rectus muscle.

Procedure:

1. Cut skin and superficial fascia.
2. Cut Lattissimus dorsi (posteriorly) and ext. oblique (anteriorly).

3. Cut Serratus posterior inferior in the posterior corner and internal oblique anteriorly (measures should be taken to save the subcostal nerve and vessels lying deep or just over the transversus).
4. Incise Lumbar fascia, push the peritoneum forwards while separating (or cutting) the fibres of transversus.
5. Lift the renal fascia, well behind the peritoneum with haemostats and incise.
6. Separate the fatty capsule (peri-renal fat) from the kidney with the fingers. Define the upper and lower poles.
7. After mobilisation, deliver the kidney into the wound.
8. Closure: Muscles are stitched in two layers. It is followed by skin suture with or without a drain.

A. Nephrectomy:

1. Renal tumours (malignant), tumours of renal pelvis will need nephroureterectomy.
2. Pyonephrosis
3. Renal tuberculosis (nephroureterectomy)
4. Hydronephrosis

Where there is massive destruction of parenchyma and the kidney is function- less. The other kidney must be functioning.)

5. Trauma: grossly lacerated with profuse haemorrhage. threatening life.

The pedicle of the kidney is defined and dealt either by mass ligation or individual ligation. The kidney pedicle clamp may be necessary.

B. Pyelolithotomy:

The kidney is drawn well forward over the wound margin so that its posterior surface is exposed. The pelvis is cleared of fat by gauze stripping. Stone/s are palpated and steadied. Incision is made in the posterior wall of the pelvis directly over the stone and radiating towards the pelvi-ureteric junction. Stone is removed by forceps or scoop.

After completion of the procedures (irrigation of pelvis and passage of a bougie down the ureter), the incision in the pelvic wall is repaired with interrupted sutures of the fine catgut.

C. Neophrolithotomy:

It is indicated when there has been previous surgery. with adhesions making approach to the pelvis difficult, The incision is made just behind and parallel to the most prominent part of the convex border of the kidney (Brodel's line).

Thermocouple regulated cooling may be required to enable the renal pedicle to be clamped.

Pyelolithotomy may be combined with Nephrolithotomy (Pyelonephrolithotomy).

30
Exposure of the Ureter and Ureterolithotomy

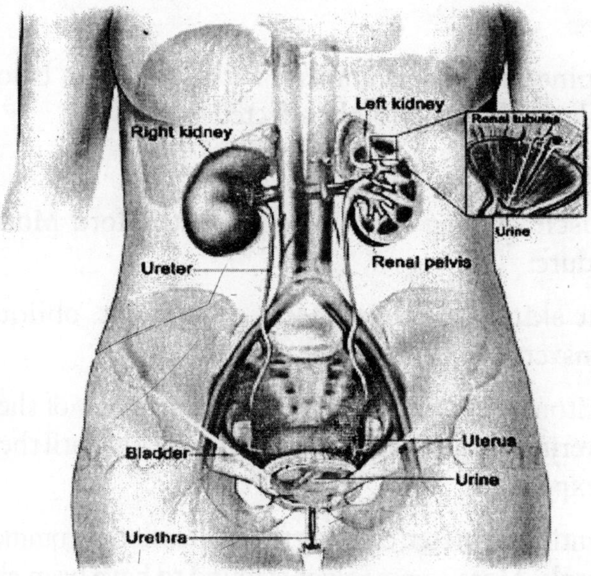

Fig. 30

Indications:

a. The stone when first seen is too large to pass naturally.
b. Gross evidence or obstruction is present or a hydronephrosis increasing.
c. Repeated attacks of colic produce no advance of the stone.

d. The stone is enlarging but not moving.

e. The urine is infected.

It is a wise precaution to carry out X-ray examination immediately prior to operation.

I. Stone Impacted in the Upper Third of the Ureter:

The incision is similar to that for exposing the kidney.

II. *Stone Impacted in the Lower Two Thirds of the Ureter,* but above the ischical spine.

Position:

Supine or semi recumbent with sand bags below the shoulder and buttock of the affected side.

Incision:

Muscle cutting iliac Incision (Rutherford Morrison). Procedure:

1. Cut skin, superficial fascia, ext. & int. oblique and transversus muscles in the same line.
2. Peritoneum is swept forwards and medially of the fascia covering the iliacus and retracted medially until the ureter is exposed.
3. Identify the ureter, crossing the bifurcation of common iliac vessels. More commonly it is found to have been elevated alongwith the peritoneum.
4. Pass a tape around the ureter, after mobilisation.
5. Palpate the stone, steady between finger and thumb (stone may be milked upwards or downwards to a convenient point for extraction).
6. Incise the ureter longitudinally over the stone.

7. Remove the stone with forceps or scoop.
8. Close the incision in the ureter with fine plain catgut suture passing through the muscular coat only.
9. Close the wound in layers with a drainage tube.

III. Stone Impacted in the Juxta Vesical or Intra-Mural Portions of the Ureter:

Position:

Supine, preferably in trendelenburg's position.

Incision:

Sub-umbilical midline incision.

Procedure:

1. After cutting the skin, linea alba etc. Peritoneum is stripped from the dome of the bladder & from the side wall of pelvis.
2. Blunt dissection between the posterior surface of the bladder and the wall of the pelvis.
3. Try to palpate the stone.

(In case of difficulty the ureter should be defined where it crosses the iliac vessels, and traced downwards. At times, bladder should be opened, ureteric orifice defined and ureteric catheter may have to be passed).

4. Remove the stone as described above.
5. Closure in layers with a drain.

31

Mastectomy

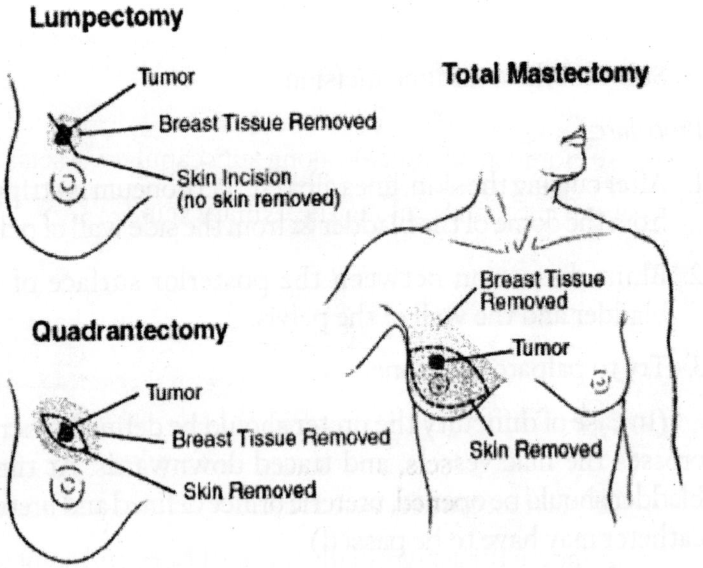

Anatomy:

Surgical anatomy:

The breast extends from 2nd to 6th rib & from sternum to anterior axillary line.

The ligaments of cooper conical projections of fibrous tissue, filled with breast tissues, apices of which is attached to the deeper layer of skin.

Areola contains:

a. sweat glands

b. sebaceous glands (glands of Montogomery) and

c. accessory mammary glands.

Arterial supply:

1. Branches from lateral thoracic (branch of axillary artery).
2. Internal mammary (perforating branches).
3. Branches from intercostal arteries.

Lymphatics:

1. Anterior (Pectoral) : lying deep to pectoralis major.
2. Posterior (Subscapular) : along subscapular vessels.
3. Lateral (Brachial) : along the axillary vein.
4. Central: within the axillary fat.
5. Apical: at the apex of axillary. immediately behind the clavicle.
6. Internal mammary group (mainly from the medial half of the breast): along the internal mammary vessels.

Simple Mastectomy Indications:

Carcinoma Breast. specially stage III & IV and sometimes in stage I & II.

Benign tumour: sero-cystic disease of Brodie.

Radical Mastectomy:

Stage I & II of Carcinoma Breast.

Structures removed:

1. Whole breast including nipple and arcola and a large portion of skin.

2. All fat and fascia from the lower border of the calvicle to the upper rectus sheath and from the sternum to the anterior border of Lattisimus dorsi.
3. Pectoralis major: sternal portion.
4. Pectoralis minor.
5. Fat fascia and lymph nodes of axilla.

The following structures should be preserved

1. The axillary vein.
2. The cephalic vein.
3. The nerve of Bell (nerve to serratus anterior).

32

Thyroidectomy

Surgical Anatomy:

Blood supply.

Arteries:

1. Superior thyroid : From external carotid (in relation to external laryngeal nerve).
2. Inferior thyroid : From thyrocervical trunk (related to recurrent laryngeal nerve).
3. Thyroidea ima : From innominate or aortic arch.

Veins:

Superior thyroid ⎤
Middle thyroid ⎦ drain into internal jugular

Inferior thyroid veins (Four) drain into innominate.

Subtotal or Partial Thyroidectomy:

1. a. Nodular goitre - toxic.

   nontoxic in view of its possible complications.

   b. Diffuse hyperplastic goitre - for cosmetic reasons.

A selective subtotal thyroidectomy is undertaken where 3/4 of the gland is removed (when normal thyroid tissue only is preserved).

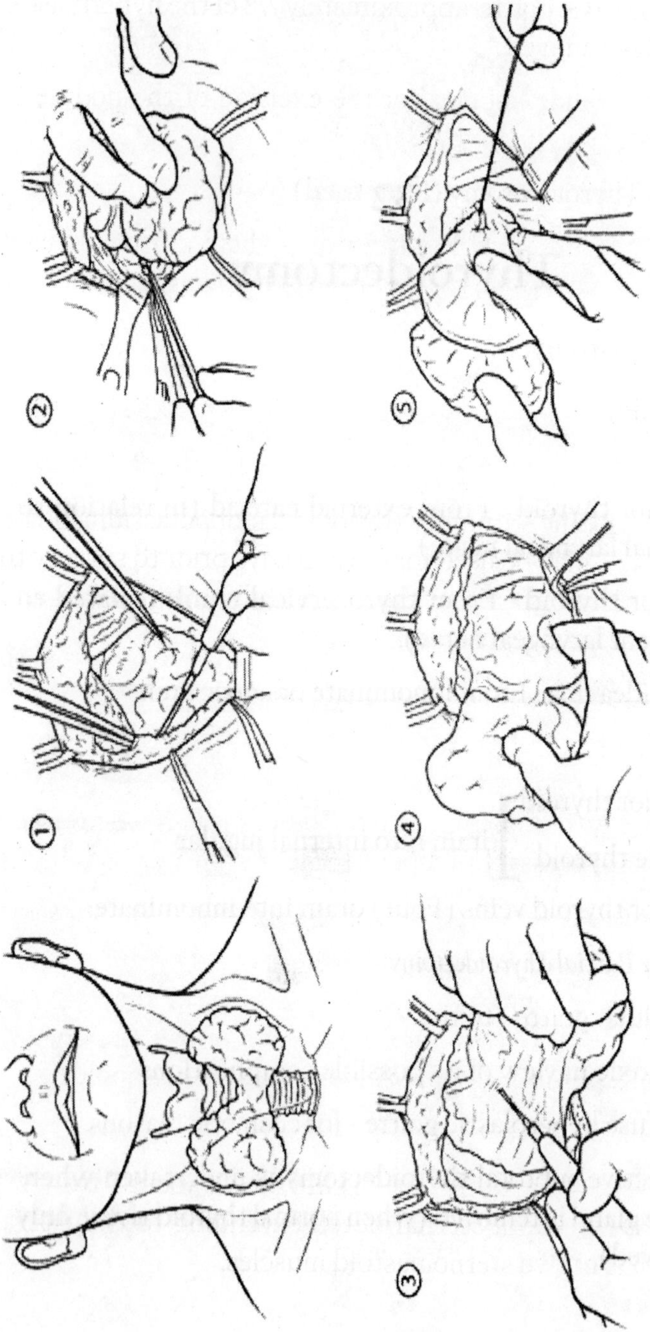

Fig. 32

II. Diffuse toxic goitre-approximately 7/8 of the hyperplastic gland is removed.

III. Toxic nodule-subtotal or the excision of the nodule is indicated.

Total Thyroidectomy (Near total)

Indicated in operable carcinoma, where a little thyroid tissue may have to he left to protect the parathyroid artery and gland.

Preparation of Thyrotoxic Patients:

Carbimazole (30-40 mg. daily) is given till the patient becomes euthyroid (takes about 8 to 12 weeks).

Lugol's iodine 30 minims (drops) t.d.s. or potassium iodide 60 mg. t.d.s. may be used for 10 to 15 days prior to surgery to reduce the vascularity of the goitre and make it softer and easier to handle.

Propranolol may be used in place of Lugol's iodine and should be continued for few days after operation.

Indirect laryngoscopy (to exclude the vocal cord palsy) : Investigations like thyroid antibodies, serum calcium are sometimes necessary preoperatively.

Anaesthesia:

General with endotracheal intubation.

Position:

Patient lies supine with sand bag under-the shoulders.

Procedure:

1. Collar incision in the line of skin crease about 3 to 5 ems above the supra sternal notch extending to the lateral borders of two sternomastoid muscles.

2. Skin incision deepen through the superficial fasical and the platysma muscle.
3. Flaps of skin, subcutaneous tissue and platysma are rellected upwards to the level of thyroid notch and downwards to the sternal notch (Joll's self-retaining , retractor may be applied).
4. Divide anterior jugular veins between ligatures.
5. Incise cervical fascia (investing layer of deep fascia) in the, midline.
6. Transverse incision of the pretracheal (infrahyoid)muscles to the carotid sheath-divided high up as ansa hypoglossi supply them from below.

   (In selected cases retraction of the muscles will suffice).
7. Mobilization of the gland: Lateral surface of the gland is cleared, middle thyroid vein (veins) divided between ligatures.
8. Muscles are retracted upwards and laterally, upper pole is delivered in the wound, cricothyroid window is opened.
9. Superior thyroid lease of vessels arc clamped between two pairs of artery forceps, applied close to the gland (to avoid injury to external laryngeal nerve). Pedicle is divided. Upper stump is doubly ligated (preferably with transfixing ligature).
10. Lower pole is delivered forwards. Inferior thyroid veins are secured.
11. The lobe is drawn forwards. Inferior thyroid artery is defined and ligated in continuity well away from the gland to prevent injury to the recurrent laryngeal nerve.
12. Isthmus is divided (after opening the space between the isthmus and trachea).

13. Ring of artery forceps around the thyroid.
14. Amount of thyroid decided and excised.
15. Cut surface stitched with catgut.
16. Haemostasis secured.
17. Other side dealt similarly.
18. Wound closure with drainage.

Complications:

I. Complication of any operation

a. General: cardiac, pulmonary, thrombotic.

b. Haemorrhage: tension haemotoma leading to respiratory obstruction. Urgent evacuation (cut the stitches) is essential.

c. Infection.

II. Damage to related anatomical structures:

a. Recurrent laryngeal nerve: unilateral or bilateral transient or permanent. Bilateral lesion may need emergency tracheostomy.

b. Injury to trachea: laryngeal oedema, respiratory obstruction.

III. Hormonal:

a. Tetany (Parathyroid insufficiency) : 2 to 5 days after operation. Usually due to vascular insufficiency to the Parathyroid.

b. Thyroid crisis.

c. Thyroid insufficiency.

d. Late recurrence of toxicity.

33
Tracheostomy

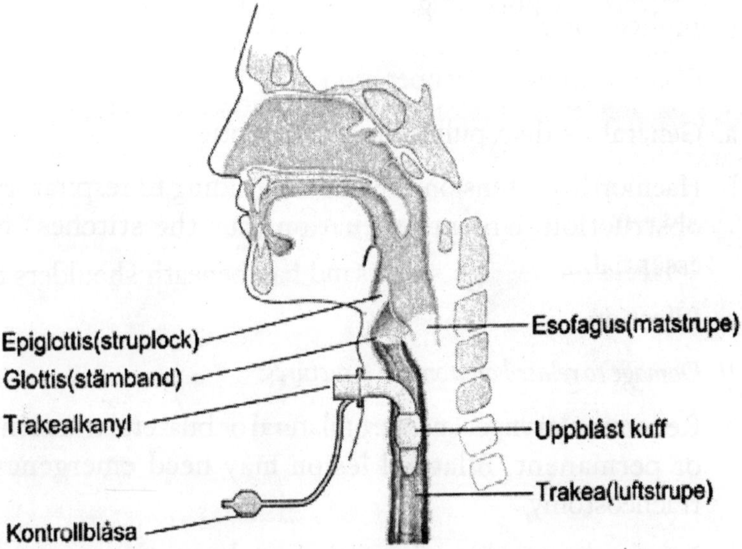

Fig. 33

Indications:

A. To relieve acute respiratory obstruction

1. Laryngeal diphtheria
2. Impaction of a foreign body
3. Oedema of the glottis
4. Bilateral recurrent' nerve injury at thyroidectomy

5. Tumours, stenosis or cut throat.

B. To improve respiratory function

a. by reducing the dead space

b. by aspiration of secretions

c. by positive pressure or assisted respiration.

1. Head injuries and coma from any other cause e.g. barbiturate poisoning.
2. Chest injuries (flail chest).
3. Bulbar type of poliomyelitis.
4. Tetanus.

Position:

Place a pillow or a small sand bag beneath shoulders to keep the neck hyperextended.

Anaesthesia:

Local anaesthesia.

Procedure:

1. Vertical incision exactly in the mid line from the upper border, of cricoid cartilage downwards for 1 and half 2 inches.

   When circumstances permit a transverse skin incision midway between the cricoid and suprasternal notch is preferable.

2. Incise skin, superficial fascia, platysma & deep fascia. may secure the anastomising veins connecting the two anterior jugulars.
3. Incise deep fascia exactly in the mid line & open the space between the strap muscles.
4. Retract the isthmus of the thyroid gland upwards or ligate & divide, if it is large.

5. Define trachea by palpating its rings & by its corrugated appearance.
6. Steady trachea by inserting cricoid hook under the cricoid cartilage.
7. Incise trachea through the 3rd or 4th rings vertically. (Sometimes oval hole is also preferred).
8. Introduce tracheal dilator.
9. Introduce tracheostomy tube & remove the dilator.
10. Tie the attached tapes of the outer tube around the patient's neck (Inner tube must be left free).
11. Place a thin veil of gauze over the tracheostomy tube.
12. If necessary, suture skin with one or two stitches.

After Treatment:

Suction of secretions are carried out as & when required. Inner tube is removed & washed in sodium bicarbonate solution every four hours.

Complications:

1. Crusting in the trachea.
2. Surgical emphysema: usually due to slipping of the tube into the tissues of the neck.
3. Mediastinal emphysema: due to low intrapleural tension.
4. Tracheal stenosis.

34
Empyema Thoracis

The treatment of empyema thoracis may be:

1. Repeated aspiration through 8th or 9th intercostal space in between mid axillary and scapular lines.
2. Intercostal drainage (under water seal).
3. Costal drainage (drainage by rib resection) : usually 2 to 2 and half inches of 8th or 9th rib between the posterior axillary and scapular lines is resected; sub-periosteally. Under water seal drainage is instituted. If possible the patient is operated in the sitting position under local anaesthesia.
4. Decortication: removal of empyema cavity.

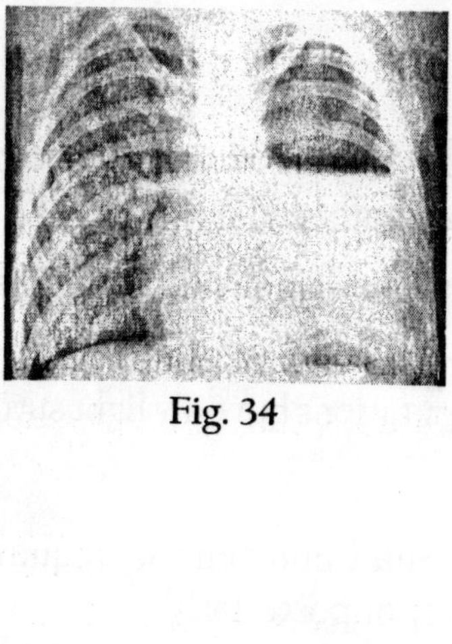

Fig. 34

35

Amputations

A. Indications:

1. Dead limb : e.g. due to:

a. Severe trauma, especially to major blood vessels.

b. Gangrene due to arteriosclerosis, thrombosis, embolism or diabetes.

2. Lethal limb : e.g., malignant tumour or gas gangrene.

3. Useless limb; The affected limb may be considered inferior to an artificial limb or to no limb at all e.g. *flail limb as a result of poliomyelitis.

   * repeatedly infected, by osteomyelitis.

B. Types

1. *Provisional:*

When primary healing is unlikely to occur because of ischaemia or infection.

a. Guillotine: All tissues are divided at the same level

b. Skin flap type: Flaps of skin and deep fascia are raised as with definitive amputations but only light suturing is employed.

2. *Definitive:*

a. End bearing: Solid bony end is' required with the scar situated anteriorly or posteriorly.

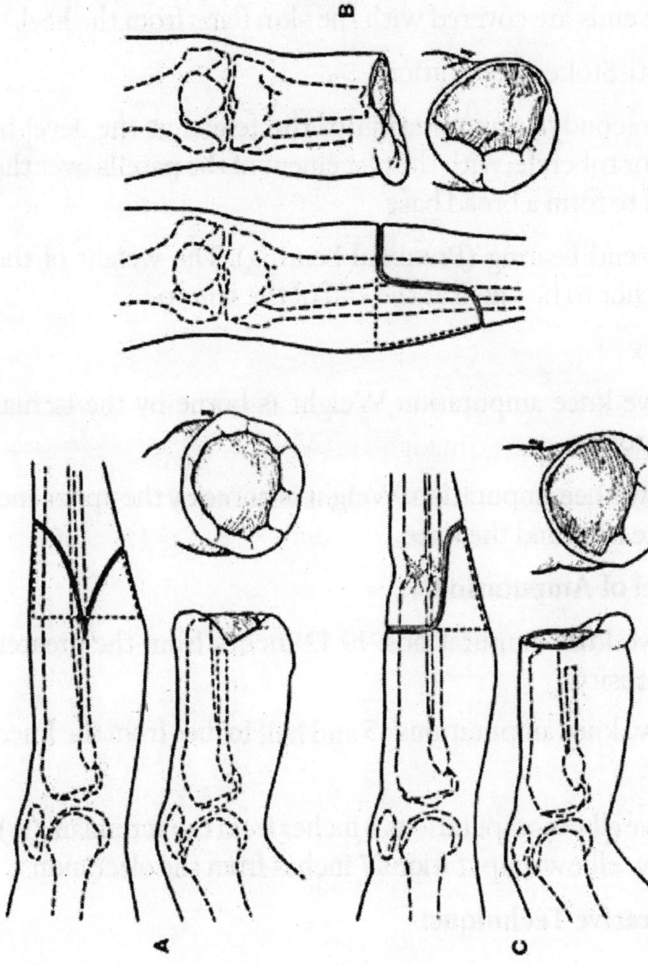

Fig. 35

Examples are:

Syme's amputations-

Tibia and Fibula are divided at the level of the ankle joint and the ends are covered with the skin flaps from the heel.

Gritti-Stokes amputations-

Supracondylar amputation of the femur at the .level of adductor tubercle, with the placement of the patella over the cut end to form a broad base.

b. Non-end bearing (Proximal bearing): The weight of the body is not to be taken at the end of the stump.

Examples:

i. Above knee amputation Weight is borne by the ischial tuberosity.

ii. Below knee amputation: Weight is borne by the upper end of the tibia and the knee.

C. Level of Amputation:

i. Above knee amputations: 10-12 inches from the greater tuberosity.

ii. Below knee amputations : 5 and half inches from the knee joint.

iii. Above elbow amputations 8 inches from the acromian. (iv) Below elbow amputations 7 inches from the olecranon.

D. Operative Technique:

1. Measure the site of amputation.
2. Avoid a tourniquet if the amputation is for an ischaemic limb.
3. Cut skin flaps and the deep fascia according to the site; too long at first and subsequently tailored. Total length of

the flap or flaps should be equal to It limes the diameter (or half the circumference) of the limb at the level of bone section.

Upper limb:

equal length of anterior and posterior flaps.

Above the knee:

longer anterior flap.

Below the knee:

longer posterior nap.

Fingers and toes:

raquet shaped incision.

Palmar or planter naps are better and should always be ample in size.

4. Divide muscles distal to the proposed site of bone section.
5. Ligate vessels as they are encountered.
6. Divide nerve above the level of proposed bone section to avoid a painful neuroma.
7. Divide the bone at the proposed site, with the help of a saw.
8. Suture opposing groups of muscles over the bone end.

Close the wound with susbcutaneous tubes and apply a pressure dressing.

E. Complications:

1. Haemorrhage, haematoma.
2. Sloughing of flaps.
3. Infection, ulceration.
4. Adherent scar.

5. Osteomyelitis and ring sequestrum.
6. Painful neuroma.
7. Phantom limb: The feeling that a patient has that his limb is still present after it has been amputated.

F. Ideal Stump:

i. The stump is well healed and conical.

ii. The scar is stable, non-tender and healthy.

iii. The skin should be freely movable both on the bone and on the subcutaneous tissue.

Prevention of transmission of human immunodeficiency virus (HIV):

All body fluids from a person infected (or suspected of being infected) with HIV should be considered potentially infectious. HIV may be transmitted: (1) by needles or sharp instruments contaminated with blood or body fluids and not properly sterilized; (2) by contact between open wounds, broken skin (for example caused by dermatitis), or mucous membranes and contaminated blood or body fluids; and (3) by transfusion of infected blood or blood products, semen donation, and skin or organ transplantation. The prevention of HIV infection requires special attention to these means of transmission as well as the strict application of aseptic routine.

Most of the small number of reported infections of health workers with HIV have resulted from injuries caused by needles (for example during recapping) and other sharp instruments. After use, disposable needles and scalpel blades should be put into a puncture-proof receptacle, preferably containing a sodium hypochlorite disinfectant. Reusable needles should also be placed in a special container of disinfectant before being cleaned and sterilized.

Surgical gloves prevent transmission of HIV through contact with blood, but there is always the possibility of accidental injury and of a glove being punctured. Thick gloves should therefore be worn when needles and sharp instruments are being cleaned. Where HIV infection is prevalent among patients, needles and instruments should routinely be soaked in a chemical disinfectant for 30 min before cleaning.

Linen soiled by a patient who is or may be infected with HIV should be handled with gloves and should be collected and transported in leak-proof bags. It should be washed with detergent for 25 min at a temperature of at least 71°C. If this is not possible, it should be soaked in a hypochlorite disinfectant before washing.

Liquid wastes, such as blood and fluids removed by suction, should be carefully poured down a drain connected to a sewer or into a pit latrine. Otherwise, they should be chemically disinfected. Solid waste should be incinerated or disposed of in a pit latrine; chemical disinfection may be a temporary expedient.

Proper sterilization of all surgical instruments and supplies is crucial in pre- venting HIV transmission. All viruses, including HIV, are inactivated by steam sterilization (autoclaving) for 20 min at 100 kPa above atmospheric pressure or by dry heat in an oven for 2 hours at 170°C.

Several points of aseptic routine applicable to members of the surgical team are also particularly relevant to the prevention of transmission of HIV:

i. Areas of broken skin and open wounds should be protected with watertight dressings.

ii. Gloves should be worn during exposure to blood or body fluids and the hands should be washed with soap and water afterwards.

iii. Frequent use of ethanol or other antiseptics on the hands and arms should be avoided, because it may lead to broken skin.

iv. Protective glasses should be worn where blood splashes may occur, as during major surgery; if the eyes are inadvertently splashed, they should be washed out as soon as possible with saline.

It should be appreciated that the whole purpose of the aseptic method is to prevent transmission of infection, and that strict attention to every detail of asepsis, with special care to avoid accidental injury during operation, is the best protection against HIV.

Fluid and electrolyte therapy, blood transfusion, and management of shock

The amount of water in the healthy body depends on the size, weight (particularly lean body mass), and sex of the individual. Body water is usually expressed as a percentage of body weight and is approximately 60% in men, 50% in women, 65% in children older than one year, and up to 75% in neonates. The water present within the cells, intracellular fluid, accounts for 40% of the body weight in men. The extracellular fluid makes up 20-25% of the body weight in men and 40-50% in neonates, and is subdivided into plasma and interstitial fluid. Physiologically, these three compartments of body water are interdependent.

Plasma contains proteins (chiefly albumin) and ions (mainly sodium, chloride, and bicarbonate). Water and electrolytes move freely between plasma (intravascular compartment) and the interstitial fluid, but plasma proteins enter the interstitial fluid only when the capillary endothelium is damaged, for example as a result of septic shock or burns. The protein in plasma is responsible for the intravascular colloid osmotic pressure, a major determinant of the movement of fluid across the capillary endothelium. Only a small proportion of the body's potassium is present in plasma, but the concentration of potassium ions is crucial to cardiac and neuromuscular function.

Interstitial fluid has an ionic composition similar to that of plasma. If there is a water deficit in the intravascular compartment, water and electrolytes pass from the interstitial compartment to restore the circulating blood volume. Electrolyte solutions, such as physiological (normal) saline and Ringer's lactate solution (Hartmann's solution), can pass into the interstitial space when they are administered intravenously. For this reason, they are effective in raising the intravascular circulating volume for only a short time if there is a deficit of fluid throughout the extracellular compartment. Blood, plasma, and colloids used as plasma substitutes, for example dextran, hydroxyethyl starch, and gelatin solutions (which are known as 'plasma expanders'), remain in the intravascular compartment longer and are therefore more effective in maintaining the circulation.

Intracellular fluid has a different ionic composition to extracellular fluid. The main cations are potassium and magnesium, with phosphates and proteins as the major anions.

After intravenous infusion, the water contained in physiological saline tends to remain in the extracellular compartment, but the water contained in glucose solutions is distributed throughout all body fluid compartments, the glucose being metabolized. Never give pure water intravenously, as it causes dangerous haemolysis.

In the normal individual, the amount of water and electrolytes excreted each day balances what is taken in in foods and fluids (Tables 1 & 2 given at the end of this Chapter). The kidney regulates, to a large degree, the volume and composition of body fluid. To a lesser degree the skin and lungs affect water losses, but do not regulate them.

Hydrogen ions (H+) and large amounts of carbon dioxide (CO_2) are produced during the normal metabolic activity of the body. The hydrogen ions are dis- charged into body fluids, and the carbon dioxide combines with water to form carbonic acid (H_2CO_3).

The body has extremely efficient mechanisms for buffering acids, but in disease these mechanisms are often disturbed. Of the buffer systems, the bicarbonate/carbonic acid system is the most important, but proteins, and especially haemoglobin, are also important as intracellular buffers. The normal plasma pH of approximately 7.4 is maintained within narrow limits through these buffering systems, through the control of carbon dioxide elimination by the lungs, and through the regulation of plasma bicarbonate (HCO3[-]) concentration by the kidney.

Changes in the volume or composition of the body fluids (which may occur before, during, or after surgery)can cause a severe physiological disturbance and should therefore be corrected promptly. The volume changes seen in surgical practice often affect the extracellular fluid. This fluid may he lost not only externally, for example through external haemorrhage, but also internally through sequestration (translocation or redistribution) into injured tissues, as in patients with burns, crush injuries, peritonitis, or an obstructed loop of the bowel. This internal redistribution of the extracellular fluid, at times referred to as fluid loss into the 'third space', is often overlooked, yet it can markedly reduce the circulating fluid volume.

Take a detailed history from the patient or from his or her relatives and make a careful examination to determine the nature and approximate amount of fluid lost; the diagnosis should be mainly clinical. The clinical state of the patient depends on the amount and rate of fluid loss, the underlying or associated disease, and the efficiency of compensatory mechanisms. Reliable tests for determining the amount of fluid lost are not available; in particular, the con- centration of sodium ions in the serum can be misleading. Nevertheless, the patient's blood can yield useful information: the blood urea concentration may be elevated if there is an uncorrected deficit of extracellular fluid, and the severity of dehydration (loss of water and electrolytes) may be indicated by the haemoglobin concentration or erythrocyte volume fraction. The dehydrated patient is usually thirsty with a dry mouth, sunken eyes, and reduced skin elasticity; the blood pressure may be low, associated with a small pulse pressure and tachycardia. If the fluid loss is acute and severe, the patient may develop hypovolaemic shock. Urinary output may be low and the relative density (specific gravity) of the urine high. If the patient is suffering fluid loss but with minimal signs, administer fluids orally, unless contraindicated; a solution of oral rehydration salts (ORS) in water is suitable for this (Tables 3 & 4). In patients with burns, oral rehydration saltsare a useful supplement to fluids given intravenously. The ideal solution to infuse is one whose composition most closely resembles that of the fluid lost. Replace the fluid already lost, administer fluid for daily maintenance, and anticipate and replace any continuing unusual losses. Remember that patients receiving fluid and electrolyte therapy, except those with diarrhoea, are not likely to pass faeces, so daily requirements must be adjusted accordingly. Table 5 given at the end of this Chapter shows the main features of the commonly available replacement fluids. In patients suffering fluid loss and showing obvious signs, it is convenient to begin replacement by infusing a balanced salt solution such as physiological saline (containing sodium chloride at 9 g/litre) or Ringer's lactate solution. In hot countries, water loss is proportionally greater than electrolyte loss, so infuse balanced salt solutions with caution and consider infusing 5% glucose (50 g/litre) as well. Insert a bladder catheter and measure the hourly urinary output and its relative density (specific gravity). Adjust the rate of infusion and the total amount of fluid in accordance with the patient's response, as indicated by the trend in the symptoms and signs, and in particular by the hourly urinary output and the jugular venous pressure. The ideal urinary output is at least 0.5 ml/kg of body weight per hour. Record clinical observations and assess the effect of therapy hourly. Establish a fluid input/output chart, and give clear, written instructions about the infusion programme; it is preferable to update these instructions every 6-8 hours rather than only once a day, as losses and requirements may change rapidly. Hypernatraemia (an excess of sodium ions in the serum, which can be confirmed by a blood test) may be caused by infusion of excessivequantities of saline or by tube feeding without sufficient water supplementation. Associated clinical fea- tures are restlessness, tachycardia, dry, sticky mucous membranes, and often an elevated body temperature. Correct hypernatraemia by salt restriction and an intravenous infusion of 5% glucose in water. Hyponatraemia may follow the intravenous infusion of large volumes of salt-free fluids, such as glucose solutions. It can also follow oral or rectal administration of large amounts of water or other salt-free fluids. It is a recognized complication of water enema in infants and children, especially in those with Hirschsprung's disease, and any form of enema in children and infants should therefore be avoided. The affected patient is lethargic and hypertensive, with tachycardia and cold extremities; oliguria or even anuria is present. Treat hyponatraemia by restricting the patient's water intake. Do not give hypertonic saline infusions in an attempt to "normalize" the level of serum sodium.

Imbalances of serum potassium concentration have more serious clinical con- sequences than those of serum sodium concentration. Potassium is crucial to cardiac and neuromuscular functions, and its level in serum (3.5-4.5 mmol/ litre) varies with the acid-base status and renal function of the individual. Hyperkalaemia may occur after severe trauma (including burns and surgical operations) and in patients suffering from acidosis, various catabolic states, and acute renal failure. Although the patient may complain of nausea, vomiting, abdominal colic, and diarrhoea, the symptoms are a poor guide to hyperkalaemia. The electrocardiogram usually has a peaked T wave, a widened QRS complex, and a depressed S-T segment; dysrhythmias are more likely than usual and may lead to cardiac arrest. Give specific treatment intravenously, in the following sequence:

i. 20 ml of a 10% (100 gllitre) solution of calcium gluconate, over a period of 20 min;

ii. 100 mmol (8.4 g) of sodium bicarbonate in solution (in an acidotic patient this will encourage the entry of potassium ions into cells);

iii. 100 ml of a 50% (500 gllitre) glucose solution, with insulin at 1 International Unit for every 5 g of glucose.

Recovery of cardiac function is usually prompt with this treatment. If the patient's hyperkalaemia is due to acute renal failure, refer the patient immediately after resuscitation, if possible. If referral is not possible, begin peritoneal dialysis.

Hypokalaemia often results from prolonged administration of diuretics or exces- sive losses of fluid through the gastrointestinal tract, for example in cases of prolonged diarrhoea or vomiting. The patient has flaccid limbs, reduced tendon reflexes, and paralytic ileus. The electrocardiogram shows a flat T wave and a depressed S—T segment. An adequate urine output (0.5 ml;kg of body weight per hour) must be established before correction of the potassium deficit is started. Potassium is given as potassium chloride mixed in the drip fluid: add 40 mmol of the salt to 1 litre of either saline or 5%glucose. Infuse this fluid very slowly so as to deliver not more than 40 mmol of potassium per hour, and estimate the serum potassium concentration after giving every 40 mmol. The bottle of fluid con- taining potassium chloride must be clearly labelled. Never give a concentrated solution of a potassium salt by direct intravenous injection.

Blood transfusion

Transfusion with whole blood is generally indicated in cases of acute, severe blood loss amounting to over 15% of blood volume. However, the decision to proceed with transfusion should be taken only after careful consideration of the risk of transfusing blood contaminated with infectious agents, including human immunodeficiency viruses.

It is not necessary to replace all lost blood with blood. To reduce the requirement for whole blood after acute blood loss, infuse plasma expanders such as dextran, hydroxyethyl starch, and gelatin solution, if available. These plasma expanders, however, cannot transport oxygen. They can also interfere with the cross- matching of blood, so blood samples should be taken before infusion.

If anaemia is recognized before surgery, it is best to investigate the cause and treat it appropriately. But in an emergency you may have to correct the anaemia by slow transfusion, preferably with packed red cells. Take particular care with haernostasis during the operation. Measure the blood loss and replace this with whole blood. If you anticipate a loss of more that 500 ml during the operation, group and cross-match donor blood in advance.

Clearly record the reasons for transfusion. Also record the history of previous transfusions, as well as any reactions to these. If the patient is a woman, record the history of any previous pregnancies, including miscarriages, stillbirths, or infants who suffered from haemolytic disease of the newborn. Finally, record the patient's current or last known haemoglobin level.

Take 10 ml of venous blood from the patient with a dry syringe, and allow it to clot in a dry, sterile specimen bottle or tube clearly labelled with the date and the patient's name, hospital number, and ward. Venepuncture may be difficult in infants, so use a heel stab instead, and allow 10-20 drops of blood to drip into a sterile tube. Except in emergencies, make requests for grouping and cross- matching of blood at least 24 hours before the proposed transfusion. This will help avoid errors and will allow time to obtain blood and carry out any tests indicated by the patient's condition.

Ideally the blood used for transfusion should match the patient's own blood group. To avoid risks to future pregnancies or transfusions, always use Rh- compatible or Rh-negative blood for premenopausal female patients. If there is difficulty in obtaining blood, especially in an emergency, apply the following rules:

Group A patient: ideally give blood group A, but you may give group O.

Group B patient: ideally give blood group B, but you may give group O.

Group AB patient: ideally give blood group AB, but you may give group A, B, or 0 (in that order of preference).

Group 0 patient: give only blood group O.

Even if these rules are followed, it is still important to cross-match the serum of the patient against the red cells of the donor (compatibility test) to make sure that the blood is safe to give.

Store blood for transfusion in a special refrigerator at 4-6 °C until the time for transfusion. There is an increased risk of sepsis if the blood is artificially warmed; it will reach room temperature as it passes down the giving set. Do not transfuse blood if it is purple, if the plasma layer is pink, or if the date of transfusion is more than 21days from the date of donation. Always use a giving set with a filter, and start transfusion slowly until about 200 ml have been given. For an anaemic patient use a slow transfusion rate throughout the procedure, but do not allow longer than 4-6 hours per unit of blood because of the risk of sepsis in blood kept at room temperature. Limit the transfusion of whole blood to 20 ml/kg of body weight for infants weighing less than 25 kg and to 10 ml/kg for neonates (up to 1 year old).

Complications

The manifestations of transfusion reactions vary, but pyrexia (at times with rigor) is common, and the patient may develop oliguria or anuria after a severe reaction. If a reaction occurs, stop the transfusion at once and investigate the cause. The reaction may be due to incompatibility between blood-group antigens and antibodies (ABO incompatibility); transfusion ofhaemolysed blood (for example blood older than 21 days); transfusion of infected blood; transfusion of blood containing allergens; accidental injection of air with the blood (causing air embolism); overloading of the circulation; or transfusion of blood containing (non-ABO) antigens or antibodies incompatible with the antibodies or antigens of the patient.

Certain diseases can be transmitted in the blood. They include malaria, syphilis, trypanosomiasis, leishmaniasis, viral hepatitis, and acquired immunodeficiency syndrome (AIDS). Always test for syphilis, and in endemic areas also make blood films to check for malaria, trypanosomiasis, and infection with Leishmania donouani. It is hoped that appropriate screening tests for viral hepatitis and for AIDS will soon be widely available.

Autotransfusion

Autotransfusion, i.e., using the patient's own blood for transfusion, is a convenient, useful, and safe procedure in cases of massive internal bleeding. The main indication for autotransfusion is a ruptured spleen or a ruptured ectopic preg- nancy, although it can also be used in the case of a large haemothorax. The blood is collected from the peritoneal (or pleural) cavity, filtered, and mixed before use with citrate to prevent coagulation.

Equipment

Specific equipment requirements are two or three sterile, D.S-litrebottles with stoppers, each containing 60 ml of 3.8% sodium citrate (38 g/litre) or 120 mlof "acid-citrate-glucose" solution (containing trisodium citrate dihydrate, citric acid monohydrate, and glucose); a large sterile funnel with eight layers of sterile gauze for filtering; and a sterile gallipot or jug.

Technique

Scoop out blood from the abdominal cavity with a gallipot (do not use a sucker), filter it through the gauze in the funnel, and allow it to drain into the collecting bottle (Fig. 2.2). Mix it gently with the anticoagulant by tilting the bottle from side to side. If any clot particles drain through, refilter the blood. Then stopper the bottle, The blood is now ready for transfusion into the patient.

Do not use this procedure for blood that has been in the abdominal cavity for more than 24 hours, or if the blood is or may be contaminated, as for example in a patient with bowel trauma.

Complications are unlikely provided that sterility is maintained throughout autotransfusion. Rarely the blood may become haemolysed or contaminated. Contaminated blood can give rise to septic shock or even septicaemia.

Shock

Shock is a useful clinical diagnosis, but it lacks a clear pathophysiological basis. Some degree of hypovolaemia is usually present, as after haemorrhage or the loss of other body fluids, for example because of acute burns. The patient suffering from hypovolaemic shock is often anxious; the pulse is rapid and thready, the blood pressure low, and the skin cool and clammy; and the extremities are often cyanotic. In addition, the patient's urinary output is reduced. Normovolaemic shock may occur as a complication of massive sepsis. In most cases its features are similar to those of hypovolaemic shock, but sometimes the patient is confused, with an increased (rather than reduced) peripheral blood flow, as indicated by warm, pink, and oedematous extremities.

Treat or control the cause of shock: arrest haemorrhage from wounds by firm pressure over a sterile dressing, and incise and drain an abscess without delay. Simultaneously begin the correction of circulatory and metabolic disturbances.

Delay in restoring the circulating volume of a patient with hypovolaemic shock can rapidly cause severe irreversible damage to the kidney and the brain. Therefore, insert a wide-bore cannula or the largest available needle (for example 14-gauge/2.0 mm) into a large vein in the cubital fossa or into the external jugular vein, and immediately start infusion of physiological saline or Ringer's lactate solution, since these fluids are usually readily available. (The infusion solution may be changed later, if necessary, ideally to the fluid that most closely resembles the fluid lost, and the infusion may be transferred to the long saphenous vein when there is time for a surgical "cut-down" at the ankle.) Elevate the patient's legs to increase venous return, but do not lower the trunk and head, as this impairs breathing. Measure and record the patient's pulse rate and blood pressure every 30 min.

Insert a catheter into the bladder to measure the hourly urinary output. This variable and the jugular venous pressure (estimated clinically) are indicators of the patient's fluid status and cardiac output (unless there is cardiac failure). Continue fluid replacement until the urinary output is at least 0.5 ml/kg of body weight per hour and the jugular venous pressure indicates adequate filling of the venous circulation.

Metabolic acidosis due to circulatory failure will subside if fluid replacement is adequate.

If no urine is draining, first check that the catheter is not blocked by measuring the circumference of the abdomen and performing bladder washout. Provided that the bladder catheter is patent, persistent anuria in a patient with restored circulation (normal blood pressure, adequate filling of the jugular veins, and pink, warm extremities) suggests acute renal failure. If possible, refer the patient immediately for further treatment; otherwise begin peritoneal dialysis.

In cases of shock due to massive sepsis (septic shock), manage the patient as outlined above, but also take a blood sample as soon as possible for a direct smear examination. Leukocytosis and immature granulocytes in the smear will support the diagnosis. Give a broad-spectrum antimicrobial drug or a combination of antimicrobial drugs selected according to the most likely organisms responsible for the sepsis. Gentamicin with metronidazole is a useful initial combination. Metronidazole may be best given as a suppository, since the preparation for intravenous injection is quite expensive.

Table 1. Average daily water exchanges (in ml) in an adult male

Loss	Tropical countries	Temperate countries
Through lungs and skin	1700	1000
In urine	1500	1500
In faeces (variable)	200	200
Total	3400	2700
Gain		
Water of oxidation	200	200
Net requirement	3200	2500

Table 2. Average daily losses of sodium and potassium (in mmol) in an adult male

Sodium	Tropical countries	Temperate countries
Urine	114	80-110
Sweat	16	0
Faeces	10	10
Total	140	90-120
Potassium		
Urine	47	60
Sweat	Negligible	0
Faeces	10	10
Total	57	70

Table 3. Mass concentration of components of a solution of oral rehydration salts (ORS)

	Component g/litre
Sodium chloride	3.5
Trisodium citrate, dihydrate a	2.9
Potassium chloride	1.5
Glucose, anhvdrouse	20.0
a Or sodium hydrogen carbonate (sodium bicarbonate)	2.5 g.
b Or glucose, monohydrate or sucrose	22.0 g, 40.0 g.

Table 4. Substance concentration of components of a solution of oral rehydration salts (ORS)

	Component mmol/litre
Sodium	90
Potassium	20
Chloride	80
Citrate *a*	10
Glucose e	111
a Or bicarbonate	30 mmol/litre.
b Or sucrose	117 mmol/litre.

Table 5. Commonly available replacement fluids

Fluid	*Ions (mmol/litre)* Na+	Cl-	K+	*Carbo-Energy hydrate content* (g/litre)	(kJ [kcalth])	Uses
Blood	140	100	4	5-8	NA	Blood loss
Physiological saline	154	154	0	0 (9 g/litre) *b*	0	Blood/extracellular fluid loss
Hartmann's solution (Ringer's solution)«	131	112	5	NA	NA	Blood/extracellular fluid loss lactate
Glucose 50 g/litre	0	0	0	50	837 [200]	Dehydration
Glucose/saline (glucose40 g/litre + sodium chloride 1.8 g/Iitre)	31	31	0	40	669 [160]	Maintenance of electrolyte and water balance
Sodium bicarbonate 84 g/litre	1000	0	0	0	0	Acute acidosis
Dextran 70 in physiological saline	144	144	0	0	0	Intravascular replacement
Polygeline	145	150	0	0	669 [160]	Intravascular replacement

a Also contains Ca2+ at 2.3 mmol/litre.

b The same as a 0.9% solution.

c Also contains Ca" at 3 mmol/litre and lactate at 28 mmol/litre. which is converted to bicarbonate and is therefore useful lor correcting acicosis. NA, not applicable

Postoperative recovery and discharge

Recovery from anaesthesia and surgery can be divided into three phases:

1. First stage recovery lasts until the patient is awake, protective reflexes have returned and pain is controlled. This should be undertaken in a recovery area with appropriate facilities. Use of modern drugs and techniques may allow early recovery to be complete by the time the patient leaves the operating theatre, allowing some patients to bypass the first stage recovery area . Most patients who undergo surgery with a local anaesthesia can be fast-tracked in this manner.

2. Second stage recovery ends when the patient is ready for discharge. You should be equipped to deal with common postoperative problems (shock, pain) as well as emergencies (haemorrhage, cardiovascular events). The anaesthetist must be contactable to help deal with problems. Protocols may be adapted to allow low-risk patients to be discharged without fulfilling traditional criteria. Mild postoperative confusion in the elderly after surgery is common. This is usually insignificant and should not influence discharge provided social circumstances permit; in fact, the avoidance of hospitalisation after minor surgery is preferred . Patients and their families should be provided with written information that includes warning signs of possible complications and where to seek help. Protocols should exist for the management of patients who require unscheduled admission, especially in a stand-alone unit.

3. Late recovery ends when the patient has made a full physiological and psychological recovery from the procedure. This may take several weeks or months and is beyond the scope of this document.

Postoperative instructions and discharge

The patient should be mobilised within 24 hours. They should be aware and encouraged to meet milestones for mobilisation, drinking and eating. This requires active involvement from both the medical and nursing teams in the immediate postoperative period. The provision of a specified dining room, with access to high calorie drinks and where meals can be taken, encourages the patient to mobilise.

All patients should receive verbal and written instructions on discharge and be warned of any symptoms that might be experienced. Wherever possible, these instructions should be given in the presence of the responsible person who is to escort and care for the patient at home.

Advice should be given not to drink alcohol, operate machinery or drive for 24 hours after a general anaesthetic . More importantly, patients should not drive until the pain or immobility from their operation allows them to control their car safely and perform an emergency stop. Procedure-specific recommendations regarding driving should be available.

All patients should be discharged with a supply of appropriate analgesics and instructions in their use. Analgesia protocols relating to minor surgery case mix should be agreed with the pharmacy. Pre-packaged take-home medications should be provided as they are convenient and prevent delays and unnecessary visits to the medicine store.

Bibliography

1. Department of Health. The NHS Plan. A Plan for Investment. A Plan for Reform. London: DoH, 2000.
2. NHS Institute for Innovation and Improvement. Better Care, Better Value Indicators. http://www.productivity.nhs.uk.
3. Department of Health NHS Modernisation Agency. 10 High Impact Changes for Service Improvement and Delivery, 2004. http://www.ogc.gov.uk/documents/Health_High_Impact_Changes.pdf.
4. Department of Health. Day surgery: Operational Guide. Waiting, Booking and Choice, 2002. http://www.dh.gov.uk/dr_consum_dh/groups/dh_digitalassets/@dh/@en/documents/digitalasset/dh_4060341.pdf.
5. NHS Institute for Innovation and Improvement. Focus On: Cholecystectomy. Coventry: NHS Institute for Innovation and Improvement, 2006.
6. Association of Anaesthetists of Great Britain and Ireland. Pre-operative Assessment and Patient Preparation – The Role of the Anaesthetist , London: AAGBI, 2010.
7. American Academy of Neurology. Practice parameter. The management of concussion in sports. Neurology. 1997; 48:581–585.
8. NHS Enhanced Recovery Partnership Programme. Delivering Enhanced recovery.

9. Helping Patients to Get Better Sooner After Surgery, 2010. http://www.dh.gov.uk/dr_consum_dh/groups/dh_digitalassets/@dh/@en/@ps/documents/digitalasset/dh_115156.

10. Ansell GL, Montgomery JE. Outcome of ASA III patients undergoing day case surgery. British Journal of Anaesthesia 2004; 92: 71–4.

11. Aldwinckle RJ, Montgomery JE. Unplanned admission rates and post discharge complications in patients over the age of 70 following day case surgery. Anaesthesia 2004; 59: 57–9.

12. Canet J, Raeder J, Rasmussen LS, et al. Cognitive dysfunction after minor surgery in the elderly. Acta Anaesthesiologica Scandinavica 2003; 47: 1204–10.

13. Davies KE, Houghton K, Montgomery JE. Obesity and day-case surgery. Anaesthesia 2001; 56: 1112–5.

14. Lewis S, Stocker M, Houghton K, Montgomery JE. A patient survey to determine how day surgery patients would like preoperative assessment to be conducted. Journal of One-day Surgery 2009; 19: 32–6.

15. Chung F, Yuan H, Yin L, Vairavanathan S, Wong DT. Elimination of preoperative testing in ambulatory surgery. Anesthesia and Analgesia 2009; 108:467–75.

16. Smith I. Emergency day surgery. Journal of One-day Surgery 2009; 19: 2–3.

17. Bhattacharyya M, Gerber B. Minimally-invasive surgical repair of ruptured Achilles tendon as a day case procedure with early full weight bearing. Journal of One-day Surgery 2007; 17: 70–5.

18. Royal College of Anaesthetists and Association of Anaesthetists of Great Britain and Ireland. You and Your

Anaesthetic. Information to Help Patients Prepare for an Anaesthetic, 3rd edn. London.

19. Castero C, Bertinato L, Baccaglini U, Drace C, McKee M. Perioperative Care Collaborative. Copenhagen: WHO European Centre for Health, 2007.

20. Association of Anaesthetists of Great Britain and Ireland. Standards of Monitoring During Anaesthesia and Recovery 4. London: AAGBI, 2007.

21. Yogendran S, Asokumar B, Cheng DCH, Chung F. A prospective randomized double-blind study of the effect of intravenous fluid therapy on adverse outcomes on outpatient surgery. Anesthesia and Analgesia 1995; 80:682–6.

22. Pavlin DJ, Pavlin EG, Fitzgibbon DR, Koerschgen ME, Plitt TM. Man- agement of bladder function after outpatient surgery. Anesthesiology 1999; 91:42.

23. Royal College of Surgeons of England. Commission on the Provision of Surgical Services. Guidelines for Day Case Surgery. London: HMSO, 1992.

24. Weidmann C, Grundy P. Day-case awake craniotomy for tumour resection. Journal of One-day Surgery 2008; 18: 45–7.

25. Hamer C, Holmes K, Stocker M. A generic process for transferring procedures to the day case setting: the Torbay hospital proposal. Journal of One-day Surgery, 2008; 18: 9–12.

26. Wilmore DW, Kehlet H. Recent advances: management of patients in fast track surgery. British Medical Journal 2001; 322: 473–6.

27. Minor surgery, a text and atlas, John S.Brown, 4th edition, 2000.

28. Basic surgical technique, R.M Kirk, 5th edition, 2002.

Notes on Spagyrics

By Dr. Debasish Kundu

Rs. 395/- US $ 21.50 Paperback

In this book author briefly discusses the principles of Alchemy with some exceptional notes on Sexual and Spiritual Alchemy.

CONTENTS: Note to the Readers, Foreword, Preface, Introduction, History of Alchemy, Spagyrics, Principles of Spagyrics, The Quest for the Quintessence, Plant Alchemy, Energetic Spagyrics, The Three Philosophical Principles, Spagyric Electro-Homoeopathy, Energy in the Organism, Herbal Medicine, Spiritual Alchemy, Sexual Alchemy, Spagyric Meditation, Hermetic Philosophy, Fermentation and Distillation of Wine Spirit, Spagyric Experiments, Explanation of Some Spagyrics Terms, Bibliography

Materia Medica and Practice of Medicine in Electro-Homoeopathy

By Dr.Debasish Kundu

Rs. 395/- US $ 21.50 Paperback

CONTENTS: Foreword, Preface, Electrohomoeopathy-An Introduction, Life History of Count Cesare Mattei, Preparation of Electro Homoeopathic Remedies, Electrohomoeopathy Formulas, Constitution and Temperament, Materia Medica of Electrohomoeopathy Medicines, Examination of the Patient, General Rules for Using the Medicines, Practice of Medicine, Points for External Application, Chief Points and their Uses, Clinical Index, Bibliography

Treatise on Spagyric Homoeopathic Pharmacy

By Dr. Debasish Kundu & Dr. Vijay Kant Agnihotri, Sr. Scientist, CSIR, Foreworded By Prof. Raffaele Pezzani, University of Padova, Italy

Rs. 395/- US $ 21.50 Paperback

It features all necessary information about the method of preparations and formulations of Zimpel, Krauss and Bernus. It is the only book which has incorporated Spagyrics formulas of Zimpel brought back from the lost fragments of time.

According to Prof. Pezzani, it is definitely a valuable guide, a friend that every Electrohomeopathy (according to Mattei) practitioner should possess. It is a must have collection for everyone.

CONTENTS: Dedication, Foreword, Preface, Spagyric Homeopathic Pharmacy, Electrohomoeopathy Formulas, Spagyrics after Zimpel, Krauss and Bernus, Medicinal Plants, Tables of Essential Oil Yielding Plants, Bibliography

Materia Medica for the New Age Man

By Dr. Debasish Kundu, Dr A.Jayasuriya, Chancellor, The Open International University, Colombo and Edited by Dr. M Ahmed, Member, Bangladesh Homeopathy Board, Dhaka

Rs. 450/- US $ 24.50 Hardbound

This is the only book which covered all therapeutic schools of Homeopathy, from Gemmotherapy, Lithotherapy, Bach flower to Spagyric Homeopathy.

CONTENTS: Foreword to the Second Edition, Introduction, Introduction to Homeopathy, Evolution of Disease, Introduction to Vital Force, Miasms, Homeopathic Pharmacy, Case Taking, Doctrine of Dosage, Therapeutic Schools of Homeotherapeutics at a Glance, Nosodes and Sarcodes, Materia Medica, Clinical Index of Homeopathic Remedies, Mother Tinctures (External Use), Do's and Don'ts for Patients, Clinical Tips for Dummies, General Index of Remedies, References

Treatise on Electro-Homoeopathic Pharmacy

By Dr. Debasish Kundu & Dr.Ajit Singh, Foreworded By Prof. Fabio R Ambrosi, Chairman, Mattei Archieves, Italy

Rs. 195/- US $ 15.50 Paperback

CONTENTS: Foreword, Preface, Introduction to Electro Homoeopathic Pharmacy, Laboratory Equipments Used in Electro Homoeopathy Pharmacy, Vehicles used in Electrohomoeopathy, Sources of Electro Homoeopthic Medicines, Collection of Medicinal Plants, Cohobation: An Extraordinary Pharmacy, Methods of Preparation of Spagyric Medicines, Quality Control Procedures, Pharmacodynamics of Electrohomoeopathy Essences, Dosages and Mode of Administration, List of Medicinal Plants Used in

Electrohomoeopathic Remedies, Appendix 1: Terminology, Appendix 2: Prescription Writing, Appendix 3: Biographies, Appendix 4: Apparatus, Bibliography

Essentials of Acupuncture

By Dr. Debasish Kundu & Prof. Choo Led Sin, Chairman, International Federation of Acupuncture, Singapore

Rs. 995/- US $ 40.00 Hardbound

The Only Book which deals with Acupuncture Anaesthesia

CONTENTS: Preface, Introduction, History of Acupuncture, Philosophy of Acupuncture, Five Elements Theory, Diagnosis in Traditional Chinese Medicine, Evaluation and Diagnosis, The Concept of Qi, Management & Research on Some Disorders, How Acupuncture Works, Acupuncture Anesthesia, Laser Acupuncture, Auriculotherapy, Atlas of Acupuncture Points, Therapeutics of Common Ailments, Therapeutics of Common Ailments, Infertility, Impotence and Acupuncture, Acupuncture in Hairfall, Does Acupuncture Hurts, Related Therapies, Explanation of Some Terms, Marmapuncture, Bibliography

Cesare Mattei's Principles of Electro Homeopathy

Interpreted & Revised By Dr. Debasish Kundu

Rs. 395/- US $ 21.50 Paperback

The classic text has been Rewritten in simple language with much needed Interpretation & Revision. In some places the original French edition has been consulted, also enriched with footnotes wherever necessary.

CONTENTS: Preface by Editor, What is Electro-Homeopathy?, Names of the Electro-Homeopathic Remedies, General Information about the Electro-Homeopathic Remedies, Sphere of Action of the Remedies in Globules, General Remarks on the Electric Liquids, Their Mode of Application, Results of Experience, Doses and Method of Administration of the Remedies in Globules, Of Diagnosis, Principles and Rules for the Selection of the Appropriate Remedy, Easy Experiments for Beginners, Catalogue of Diseases Cured by Electro-Homeopathy, Appendix

Stepping Stones to Electo-Homoeopathy (Count Mattei's System of Medicine)

By A J L Gliddon(Original Edition with Vitiation of Blood and Lymph Theory)

Rs. 395/- US $ 21.50 Paperback

A brief insight into the discovery of electro homeopathy together with a rational explanation of the principles involved and the proposed medicines.

CONTENTS: Introduction , The Human Body, Count Mattei's Theories, Symptoms of Disease, The Electro-Homceopathic Remedies, The Globule Remedies, The Electricities, External Use of Electricities, External Use of Globules, Baths, Compresses, etc., How to Select the Remedies, How to Determine the Dose, Dilutions, Dry Globules, Table of Doses, Minute Doses, Effects of the Remedies, Other Hygienic Helps, Diet, Dress, Pure Air, etc.

Essentials of Trace Elements & Biochemic Medicine

By Prof. Dr. Debasish Kundu, Edited By Prof. Seyed Farzin Hassanzadeh Salehian Ph.D. (Iran)

Rs. 350/- US $ 19.00 Paperback

Cell Salts or Bioplasgens have always been considered an important part of healing in Homeopathy and Spagyrics. This book contains all essential materials concerning Trace Elements & Bioplasgen and their relationship with Spagyrics, Clinical Materia Medica with useful suggestions.

CONTENTS: Preface, Introduction to Trace Elements & Bioplasgens, The Functions of The Cell, Astrology and Bioplasgens, Minerals, Trace Elements, Materia Medica of the Bioplasgens, Bio-combinations, Bibliography

A Textbook on Food, Nutrition and Dietetics

By Dr. Debasish Kundu Editor Dr. Malik A.K. Awan Ph.D. (London), Associate Editor Prof. Seyed Farzin Hassanzadeh Salehian Ph.D.(Iran)

Rs. 495/- US $ 20.00 Paperback

CONTENTS: Preface, Relationship between Food, Nutrition & Health, History of Nutrition, Functions of Food, Digestion of Food, Food and Nutrition, Nutrition, Diet & Development, Nutrition & Diet Therapy, Nutrition for Infants, Children, Adults, Women and Elderly, Ideal Diet Plan, The Food Pyramid, Therapeutic Diet, Bibliography

Notes on MJT (Forensic Medicine & Toxicology)

By Dr. Debasish Kundu Ph.D. Assisted By Dr. Ravi Justin Raj NMD, LLB Edited By Dr. Malik A.K. Awan B.S., M.S. (Psychology), D.C.L., D.D. (U.S.A.), Ph.D. (London)

Rs. 550/- US $ 22.00 Paperback

CONTENTS: Part I: Forensic Medicine: Dedication , Preface , Introduction, Scope of Forensic Medicine, Aspects of Identification, Medico-legal Aspects of Death, Investigation of Death, Death by Asphyxia, Medico-legal Aspects of Injuries, Investigation of Wounds, Medico-legal Aspects of Sex Crimes, Medico-legal Aspects of Abortion, Forensic Pathology, Forensic Entomology, Radiation Poisoning, Medico-legal Sections in IPC, Cr PC, AND IE A, Part II: Toxicology: Introduction to Toxicology, General Approach to a Victim of Poison, Clinical Toxicology Laboratory, Practical Aspects of Analytical Toxicology, Toxicants of Public Health Hazard, Medical Toxicants, Environmental Toxicants, Abuse of Drugs, Natural Toxicants, Annexure I: Preparations of Reagents, Annexure II: Apparatuses, Annexure III: Glossary of Terms Used, Annexure IV: Abbreviations Used, Bibliography

Notes on Minor Surgery

By Dr. Debasish Kundu Ph.D. Guided & Edited by Dr. A.K. Banerjee M.B.B.S., M.D. (U.S.A.)

Rs. 395/- US $ 21.50 Paperback

CONTENTS: Part-I: Preface, Acharya Sushruta, Basic Surgical Procedures, Surgery of Some Common Conditions, Part II: Sterilisation, Suture Materials, Nomenclature of Operations, Planning for Operation, Anaesthesia,Operative Surgery, Postoperative Complications, Abscess Drainage, Venesection (Cut Down), Skin Grafting, Circumcision, Vasectomy, Hyderocele, Inguinal Hernia, Strangulated Inguinal Hernia, Femoral Hernia, Umbilical Hernia, Appendicetomy,

Abdominal Incisions, Peptic Ulcer, Vagotomy, Gastrojejumnostomy, Partial Gastrectomy, Closure of Perforated Peptic Ulcer, Right Hemicolectomy, Colostomy, Cholecystectomy, Choledocholithotomy (Supraduodenal), Spleenectomy, Lumbar Sympathectomy, Haemorrhoidectomy, Suprapubic Cystostomy, Prostatectomy, Exposure of Kidney , Exposure of the Ureter and Ureterolithotomy, Mastectomy, Thyroidectomy, Tracheostomy, Empyema Thoracis, Amputations, Bibliography

Principles and Practice of Naturopathy

By Dr. Debasish Kundu Editor Dr. Malik A. K. Awan Ph.D. (London) Associate Editor Prof. Sayed Farzin Hassanzadeh Salehian Ph.D.(Iran)

Rs. 750/- US $ 30.00 Paperback

CONTENTS: Foreword, Preface to the First Edition, Preface to the Third Edition, Naturopathy: Its Principles & Pioneers, Physiology, Food and Nutrition, Hygiene and Sanitation, Biology, Herbology, Medicinal Plants, Magnet Therapy, Yoga and Meditation, Massage Therapy, Medical Gymnastics, Chemistry, Bacteriology, Toxicology, Pathology, Osteology, Neurology, Ethics, Hydro Therapy and Helio Therapy, Colour Therapy, Fasting and Diet, Mud Therapy and Fango Therapy, Acupressure, Aromatherapy, Reflexology, Iridology, Vitamins and Balanced Diets, Bibliography

Diseases of Women (Adopted from Margaret Seifert's Krankheiten Der Franen)

By Dr. Shefalika Kundu, Edited By Dr. Debasish Kundu & Dr. Sudeshna Kundu

Rs. 350/- US $ 19.00 Paperback

The book is intended as a handbook on diseases of women with their Electrohomeopathic treatment. Besides an update on the literature on Contraception using Spagyrics , entirely new topics Anatomy of Uterus and Stages of development in Pregnancy are added.

CONTENTS: Preface to the Second Edition, Foreword to the First Edition, Preface, Introduction, Anatomy and Physiology of Sexual Organs of Women, General View of Treatment, Diseases and Their Treatment, Hygienic Care of the Body and Toilet, Anatomy of Uterus in Pregnancy, Notes on Various Diseases, Family Planning, Contraception in Electrohomoeopathy,Diet, Index of Diseases Discussed, Bibliography

Lectures on Materia Medica & Therapeutics

By Dr. H. D. Banerjee, Foreworded By M V Mattei, Thoroughly Revised & Edited By Prof. Dr. Debasish Kundu

Rs. 225/- US $ 18.00 Paperback

CONTENTS: Preface to the Third Edition, Preface to the Second Edition, Foreword to the First Edition, Introduction, On Electro-Homoeopathic Principles, On Principles of Orthodox School, On Homeopathic Principles , On Objections to Electro-Homoeopathy, Chemical Analysis of the Remedies, Dynamisation of the Remedies, On Minute Doses, On Frequency of the Doses, Purgatives in Electro-Homoeopathy, On Prescription Writing, Materia Medica & Therapeutics, On Therapeutics of the Remedies

Principles & Art of Cure in Electrohomeopathy

By Prof. Dr.Debasish Kundu Ph.D.

Rs. 195/- US $ 15.00 Paperback

CONTENTS: Introduction to Electrohomeopathy, Philosophy, The Discoverer, Principles of Nature, Introduction to Electrohomeopathy Medicines, The Iris science, Sources and preparation of Electrohomeopathy Medicines, Cohobation, Spagyric Tinctures, Classification of Electrohomeopathy Medicines, Classification, Preparation and Therapeutics uses of Electrohomeopathy Medicines, Potentisation of Electrohomeopathy Medicines and Electric fluids, Preparation and Therapeutic uses of Ointments and Lotions, Points for application Electric Fluids, Ointments and Lotions, Plain talks on using the medicines, Potentisation and Bio-Magnetism, The Similia of Electrohomeopathy, The Scientific basis of Electrohomeopathy System of Medicine, World's present day need of Electrohomeopathy, Clinical Index.

A Clinical Treatise on Cancer

By Prof. Dr.Debasish Kundu Ph.D. Foreworded By Dr. B.B. Upreti, Ph. D. General Secretary, All Nepal Electro-Homeo Medical Association, Hetauda, Nepal

Rs. 195/- US $ 15.00 Paperback

CONTENTS: Introduction, The Increase of Cancer and it's Causes, The Treatment of Cancer, Diet for Patients, Hygienic Care of the Patients

CONTENTS: Foreword, Preface, Part 1: Introduction to Spagyric Medicine, History of Alchemy, Principles of Spagyrics, The Simila of Alchemy, Difference Between Homoeopathy and Spagyric Homoeopathy, Botanical Consciousness in Spagyrics, Micronutrients and Spagyrics, Alchemy and the Zodiac Connection, How Spagyric Medicines Work, Alchemy and Spagyrics, Spagyrics : The Future in Medicine, Part 2: Pharmacy in Plant Alchemy, Pharmaceutical Process, Laboratory Apparatus, Vehicles Used in Plant Alchemy, Sources of Medicines, Preparation of Spagyric Essence, Spagyric Essence by Cohobation Method, Phytochemical Analysis of Plants, Different Spagyric Methods, Quality Control Procedures, Safety Measures in Laboratory, Doctrine of Dosage, Medicinal Plants, Terminology, Appendix, Bibliography

Mysticism, Romance & Secrets of Count Cesare Mattei (With Properly Transcripted Secret Formulas)

By Prof. Dr. Debasish Kundu , Ph.D. (U.S.A.)

Printed on Art Paper, USD ($) 40.00 Hard Bound

It is the Bible of Mattei Electrohomoeopathy : covering the true life of Cesare Mattei and properly transcripted Empirical Formulas & Secret Pharmacy of Electrohomoeopathy, incl. Medicinal Plants Used by Cesare Mattei.

Contributors-Prof. Raffaele Pezzani, University of Padova, Italy, Dr. Fabio R. Ambrosi, University of Sapienza, Rome, Italy, Prof. El Akrem Hayouni, University of Manouba, Tunisia, Allesandro Rapparini, Vice Pres., Archivio Museo Cesare Mattei, Bologna, Italy, Prof. Peter Morrell, Formerly Honorary Research Associate, History of Medicine, Staffordshire University, U.K., Dr. Terry Mitchell, Alchemist & Director, Phylak GmbH, U.K., Willow Morningsky, Spagyrist & Psychologist, Southern Oregon University, Ashland, Oregon, U.S.A. etc.

CONTENTS: Introduction, Dedication, Note to the Readers, Acknowledgements, Alchemist's Prayer, Preface, The Castle of Love, The Mystery Unveiled, Emerald Tablet of Cesare Mattei, Mysticism & Romance of Cesare Mattei, Electro Homoeopathy Pharmacology, Medicinal Plants Used by Cesare Mattei, Glossary of Pharmacological Terms, Bibliography

For Further Information and Ordering:
Originals/Low Price Publications
A-6, Second Floor, Nimri Commercial Centre,
Ashok Vihar Phase-4, Delhi - 110 052 (India)
Tel.: +91 11 2730 2453 Fax: 011 4706 1936
Mobile: 98100-12366
Website: www.Lppindia.com,
e-mail: info@Lppindia.com
info@Lbopub.com